Gerotechnology: Research and Practice in Technology and Aging

A Textbook and Reference for Multiple Disciplines

David Burdick, PhD, is Associate Professor of Psychology and Coordinator of Gerontology at the Richard Stockton College of New Jersey. He received his BA in psychology and environmental studies from Alfred University (1977), his master's (1980) and doctoral (1983) degrees in geropsychology from the University of Notre Dame, and was a Postdoctoral Fellow in Applied Gerontology with the Gerontological Society of America (1984). He is a Fellow of the Association for Gerontology in Higher Education (AGHE), a former member of AGHE's Executive committee, and an active member of several AGHE committees. Dr. Burdick is also a Fellow of the Gerontological Society of America (GSA) and Co-convener of GSA-TAG (Formal Interest Group on Technology and Aging). He serves on the editorial board of the Intergenerational Programming Quarterly and co-directs Stockton's Democracy Dialogues Project funded by AAC&U, designed to improve community engagement among students and faculty at the college. Dr. Burdick has taught a course on aging and technology since 1987.

Sunkyo Kwon, PhD, is Director of the Applied Gerontology Graduate Program at Sookmyung University, Seoul, South Korea. He has been involved in numerous ventures related to information and communication technology, both in professional service and gerontological research. He earned bachelor's degrees at Yonsei University (Republic of Korea), and the University of Maryland; a Dipl-Psych at the Institute of Psychology, Technical University Berlin; and a doctorate degree at the Free University Berlin. Dr. Kwon has held multiple research positions at the Free University Berlin, at the Humboldt University Berlin Department of Geriatrics Research and Institute for Rehabilitation Sciences, and at the Institute for Health Sciences/Public Health, Technical University Berlin. He also served a three-year term as research consultant (qualitative and quantitative methods) at the Berlin Center of Public Health, an organization affiliated and supported by Berlin's three comprehensive universities (Free University Berlin, Humboldt University Berlin, Technical University Berlin). He is current co-convener of the GSA-TAG (Formal Interest Group on Technology and Aging).

Gerotechnology: Research and Practice in Technology and Aging

A Textbook and Reference for Multiple Disciplines

David C. Burdick,
PhD

Sunkyo Kwon,
PhD

Springer Publishing Company

Springer Publishing Company, Inc.
11 West 42nd Street, 15th Floor
New York, NY 10036

Acquisitions Editior: Sheri W. Sussman
Production Editor: Jeanne Libby
Cover design by Joanne Honigman

04 05 06 07 08 / 5 4 3 2 1

Library of Congress Cataloging-in-Publication Data

    Gerotechnology : research and practice in technology and aging / edited by David C. Burdick and Sunkyo Kwon.
      p. ; cm.
    Includes bibliographical references and index.
    ISBN 0-8261-2516-6 (alk. paper)
    1. Older people—Care—Technological innovations. 2. Older people—Care—Technological innovations—Moral and ethical aspects. 3. Self-help devices for people with disabilities. 4. Geriatrics—Technological innovations. 5. Gerotechnology—Technological innovations.
    [DNLM: 1. Geriatrics. 2. Research—methods. 3. Technology—trends—Aged. 4. Computers. 5. Self-Help Devices. WT 20 G377   2004] I. Burdick, David C. II. Kwon, Sunkyo.

RA564.8.G4725   2004
618.97'03—dc22   2004017711

Printed in the United States

Contents

SECTION C: Assistive Technology in the Home and Environment

SECTION D: Models, Prototypes, and Specific Applications of Gerotechnology

SECTION E: Cautions, Integration, and Synthesis

Tables and Figures

About the Authors

Ann E. Benbow, PhD, is Chief Consultant and former Director of Adult Learning and Technology at the SPRY Foundation in Washington, D.C. She has been Principal Investigator of an NSF-funded project with the OASIS Institute: *Science Across the Generations* and an intergenerational project on high blood pressure supported by the National Heart, Lung, and Blood Institute. She earned a BS in Biology from St. Mary's College of Maryland, an MEd in Science Education, and a PhD in Curriculum and Instruction from the University of Maryland.

Heather Cameron, PhD, received her PhD in Social and Political Thought from York University, Canada (2002). She was the coordinator of the architecture and styles of life subproject of Sentha (Technical University Berlin) from 2001 to 2003. Her current research interests include how new surveillance technologies transform housing public space and how these technologies are resisted.

Neil Charness, PhD, received his BA (1969) in Psychology from McGill University and his MS (1971) and PhD (1974) in Psychology from Carnegie Mellon University. He is currently Professor of Psychology at the Florida State University and a Research Associate at the Pepper Institute on Aging and Public Policy (FSU). He has received grants related to age, expertise, and human factors from a variety of public and private foundation sources in the U.S., Canada, and Germany. He has published over 70 journal articles and book chapters related to aging, human factors, and technology, and has coedited three recent books on gerotechnology. He is a Fellow of the Canadian Psychological Association, the American Psychological Association (APA) (Division 20), the American Psychological Society (APS), and the GSA.

Hans-Liudger Dienel, Dr. Phil, is Acting Director of the Center for Technology and Society at the Technical University Berlin, Germany. He holds academic degrees both in engineering and social sciences. Dr. Dienel is coprincipal investigator of one of the largest-scale research projects in Germany on applied technology for senior citizens' everyday lives (Sentha: www.sentha.tu-berlin.de). Dr. Dienel is a prolific writer and has edited two volumes on new products for older adults.

Katharina V. Echt, PhD, holds positions as Assistant Director of the Emory Center for Health in Aging and as research scientist at the Atlanta Veterans Administration Rehabilitation R & D Center. She received a Bachelor's degree in Psychology at Jacksonville University and a PhD in Life-span Developmental Psychology and Gerontology at the University of Georgia.

Arthur D. Fisk, PhD, received a PhD in Experimental Psychology from the University of Illinois in 1982. He is currently Professor and Coordinator of the Engineering Psychology Program at Georgia Institute of Technology. He is a member of several scientific societies including: APA, GSA, Human Factors and Ergonomics Society (HFES), and Psychonomic Society. He is a Fellow of APA and of the HFES, a past president of the HFES, and a past president of the APA's Division of Applied Experimental and Engineering Psychologists. He has served as Editor of the scientific journal Human Factors, and is on the editorial board of several scientific journals.

James L. Fozard, PhD, has a long career of research on aging and development of national programs of long-term health care targeted toward older people for the U.S. Department of Veterans Affairs. Currently President of the Florida Gerontological Research and Training Services located in Palm Harbor, Florida, he is best known for work with longitudinal studies of aging including the VA Normative Aging Study and the National Institute on Aging Baltimore Longitudinal Study, which he directed for 13 years. A founding member of the International Society for Gerontechnology, he has contributed over a dozen chapters and articles to the rapidly growing literature in this interdisciplinary field. Author of over 160 articles and chapters, Fozard was a member of the faculty of The Johns Hopkins University School of Hygiene and Public Health for 10 years and the Psychiatry Department of Harvard Medical School for 12 years. He received his PhD in experimental psychology from Lehigh University and did his post-doctoral training at the Massachusetts Institute of Technology.

Anthony P. Glascock, PhD, is currently Professor of Anthropology and Director of the Center for Applied Neurogerontology at Drexel University.

His current research interests focus on the use of technology to improve the quality of life of older adults by allowing them to remain in their own residences. This interest grew out of extensive research on home health care conducted over the last decade in Ireland, Canada, and the United States. He has published over 50 articles and book chapters, and his latest book, *The Aging Experience: Diversity and Commonality Across Cultures* was awarded the Richard Kalish Innovative Publication Award presented by the Behavioral and Social Science Section of the Gerontological Society of America. He is President of Behavioral Informatics, Inc., a member of the Board of Directors of Living Independently, Inc. and holds three patents (two U.S., one Canadian) on a behavioral monitoring system.

Joy Hammel, PhD, OTR/L, is an occupational therapist who holds a BA from the University of Wisconsin-Madison, an MA in Education/instructional technology from San Francisco State University, and a PhD in educational psychology from the University of California at Berkeley. She is currently Assistant Professor in Occupational Therapy and Disability Studies at the Department of Occupational Therapy/Disability and Human Development, University of Illinois at Chicago.

Geoffrey Ho, MSci, obtained an MSc in Psychology at the University of Calgary, studying skill acquisition in visual search in an elderly population, an area where he has coauthored a number of papers and conference presentations. He subsequently did an internship at Honeywell Labs in Minneapolis, working on a variety of human factors projects. Currently he is in the PhD program at Calgary.

Penelope M. Keyl, PhD, is a chronic disease epidemiologist with a background in mathematics. She retired from the Department of Emergency Medicine at The Johns Hopkins School of Medicine in 2001 as an Associate Professor and is currently active as a consultant. Dr. Keyl was Director of the Traffic Accident Research Unit at B. C. Research, Vancouver and at The University of Calgary School of Medicine prior to coming to the U.S. in 1980. In the U.S., she has been principal- or co-investigator on several studies focusing on injury prevention and control.

David M. Kutzik, PhD, is Associate Professor of Sociology and Associate Director of the Center for Applied Neurogerontology at Drexel University, Philadelphia. Prior to joining Drexel in 1989, Dr. Kutzik was Director of Core Behavioral Research at the Polisher Institute of the Philadelphia

Geriatric Center. He is a principal of Behavioral Informatics, chiefly responsible for the development of patent protectable technologies for automated monitoring and evaluation of routine daily activities, for which he has received patents in the U.S. and Canada.

Jason Laberge, BSc, is a student in the MSc program in Experimental Psychology at the University of Calgary. He obtained his BSc in Psychology from Calgary in 1999 and has worked in a variety of labs at the university conducting research on human-computer interaction, transportation human-factors, computer supportive cooperative work, and cognitive aging.

Gari Lesnoff-Caravaglia, PhD, is Professor at the School of Health Sciences, Ohio University. She received her PhD at the University of California at Los Angeles (UCLA). Dr. Lesnoff-Caravaglia was the founder of the formal interest group "Technology and Aging" of the GSA, which she convened for nine years. Among many others, she has been the editor of the International Journal for Technology and Aging.

Christopher B. Mayhorn, PhD, is an Assistant Professor in the Ergonomics/ Experimental Psychology program at North Carolina State University. He earned his BA at The Citadel, and an MS and PhD at the University of Georgia. His current research activities and interests are in aging and applied cognition.

Heidrun Mollenkopf, PhD, received her DrPhil in Sociology from the Free University of Berlin in 1995. She has been the German delegate in the EU COST A5 programme "Ageing and Technology," and was a member of the European Commission's ETAN (European Technology Assessment Network) expert working group (DG XII). Since 1997, she has been a Senior Researcher at the German Centre for Research on Ageing (DZFA) at the University of Heidelberg, Department of Social and Environmental Gerontology. Since January 2000 she has been principal investigator and co-ordinator of the international MOBILATE (Enhancing Outdoor Mobility in Later Life) project, funded by the European Commission. She has authored numerous publications on aging and technology.

Roger W. Morrell, PhD, is Director of Research at GeroTech Corporation in Reston, Virginia. He has served as a consultant to many government agencies and private businesses related to the interests of older adults, including the National Institute on Aging, the National Library of Medicine, SPRY Foundation (the research and education arm of the National Committee for the Preservation of Social Security and Medicare), SeniorThinking.com, The Medical University of South Carolina, The National Democratic Women's Club, Practical Memory Institute, and ARINC. Dr. Morrell received his PhD in 1992 from the University of Georgia. He has published numerous articles, book chapters, and technical reports concerning older adults' use of electronic technology, and he has spoken at many conferences concerning older adults both in the U.S. and abroad. He is editor of the book *Older Adults, Health Information, and the World Wide Web.*

Mary Hamil Parker, PhD, is Managing Director, MKHP Associates, LLC. Dr. Parker was the principal investigator of the SBIR Research project that developed the Palliative Care Training Program. She also is the principal investigator of the Fox and Samuels Foundation grant project that is validating the Palliative Care Training program methods in training health care staff in New York City. She received a PhD in Public Administration from The Johns Hopkins University in 1978. She is Coconvener of the GSA Formal Interest Group on Technology and Aging (GSA-TAG).

Alexander Peine, MSc, is a research fellow with the research group "Sentha—Everyday Technology for Senior Households" (funded by the Deutsche Forschungsgemeinschaft since 1997) that is coordinated at the Centre for Technology and Society at the Technical University of Berlin. He graduated from TU Delft with an MSc (Dutch equivalent of the Dipl-Ing). Subsequently, he worked for the Institute for Ecological Economy Research in Berlin.

George W. Rebok, PhD, is a professor in the Department of Mental Health of The Johns Hopkins University. He began his career with a BA in Psychology (magna cum laude) at Muhlenberg College, and master's and doctoral degrees at Syracuse University in Life-span Developmental Psychology. His current research includes studies on memory interventions with older adults and the effects of aging and dementia on driving and other everyday functional tasks, including the benefits of physical activity on memory, using CD-ROM based multimedia technology. Dr. Rebok is a Fellow of the APA and the GSA. Currently, he is principal investigator of a multi site NIA grant for a clinical trial of cognitive intervention for older adults, and is an investigator for an NIA-funded study of pilot aging and aviation safety.

Wendy Rogers, PhD, is a professor in the Engineering and Experimental Psychology Programs, School of Psychology, at the Georgia Institute of Technology. She received her BA from the University of Massachusetts-Dartmouth, and her MS (1989) and PhD (1991) from Georgia Institute of Technology. Her research interests include skill acquisition, human factors, training, and cognitive aging. She has published extensively in the field of human factors and cognitive aging (over 60 journal articles and book chapters), and serves on the editorial boards of Psychology and Aging, Experimental Aging Research, Ergonomics in Design, and Human Factors. She is Past President and Fellow of Division 21 (Applied Experimental and Engineering Psychology) and a Fellow of Division 20 (Adult Development and Aging) of the APA. She also served as an at-large member of the Executive Council of the HFES.

Dory Sabata, OTD, has both academic training and expertise in maximizing everyday life activities or "occupational performance" to support aging in place. Currently at the University of Southern California, she is an instructor for online courses in home modifications, is a key member of the university gerotechnology initiative, is involved with an AoA funded project called Caregiver Adaptations to Reduce Environmental Stress (CARES), and is on the Archstone Foundation Steering Committee for California Fall Prevention. In 2002, she earned a PhD in Occupational Therapy from Washington University in St. Louis. She completed her BA in Gerontology and Psychology from Southwest Missouri State University in 1995.

Charles (Chip) Scialfa, PhD, is a Professor of Psychology at the University of Calgary (Canada). Dr. Scialfa earned his PhD at the University of Notre Dame and has directed Calgary's Perceptual and Cognitive Aging Lab since 1989. His current research program has several facets, including the effects of distraction on driving performance, usability and web navigation, visual search deficits in older individuals, and the role of eye movements and the "useful field of view" in explaining age-related change in visual processing. He has also been a member of the National Academy of Science's Steering Committee on Technology and Adaptive Aging.

Kathleen A. Smyth, PhD, is an Associate Professor and Acting Director of the Division of Health Services Research in the Department of Epidemiology and Biostatistics, Case Western Reserve University (Case) School of Medicine. She is also Associate Director and Director of the Caregiving Research Program at the Case/University Hospitals of Cleveland University Memory and Aging Center. She received her BA from Ursuline College (1967) and her MA (1973) and PhD (1984) from Case. Her research interestes include the correlates and impacts of family caregiving in dementia and the use of computer-mediated communication to provide support and information to family caregivers. She has published over 50 articles and book chapters focused primarily on dementia and caregiving, and is a Fellow of the Gerontological Society of America. Her work in computer-mediated support for caregivers has been recognized with one of the first National Information Infrastructure Awards and an Ameritech/National Council on the Aging Innovations in Communications Technology Award.

Binh Q. Tran, PhD, is an Assistant Professor in the Department of Biomedical Engineering and is the Director of the Cardio-Pulmonary Research Lab (CPRL) at The Catholic University of America. His major research and academic interests pertain to the areas of cardiac and pulmonary mechanics, biomedical imaging, biomedical instrumentation, home care technologies, and home health care. He received BS and MS degrees in Mechanical Engineering from the University of California at San Diego and from San Diego State University, respectively, and a PhD in Biomedical Engineering from the University of Iowa.

K. Victor Ujimoto, PhD, is a Professor of Applied Sociology, University of Guelph, and an Adjunct Professor of Human Factors and CRM in the Commercial Aviation Management Program, University of Western Ontario. He obtained his BSc in Mathematics and Physics from the Royal Military College of Canada and MA and PhD degrees in Applied Sociology from the University of British Columbia. He is currently involved in several national and international human factors research projects related to the effects of age, national culture, and shift-work on flight safety and crew performance in highly technical systems. He is a member of the Canadian Aeronautics and Space Institute, the Association of Aviation Psychologists, the Aerospace Systems Technical Group, the HFES, the GSA, and the Canadian Association on Gerontology. He was on the editorial board of the International Journal of Technology and Aging from 1988 to 1992.

James Watzke, PhD, is Research Head of Product Evaluation at the Dr. Tong Louie Living Laboratory, a full-scale simulation research facility under the Health Technology Research Group, Technology Centre, British Columbia Institute of Technology (BCIT). He obtained his undergraduate degree at the University of California, Berkeley, and his PhD at the University of Lund, Sweden. His research is on ways to make environments and products work better for older adults and persons with disabilities. He has published and presented papers extensively in assorted North American and international forums. He is founder of I-AGE, a private company that helps clients to solve problems related to environmental design and technology, as well as to provide measures to enhance quality of life for older adults and persons with disabilities.

Foreword:
Timeless Technology for All Ages

One of the main goals of this book on technology and aging has been the coverage of material that would stand the test of time. That is, we had the ambition to produce a useful and coherent collection of writings that would not become quickly obsolete due to rapid developments in technology. Anyone familiar with the inexorable march of new technology and the growing interest in research in gerontechnology/gerotechnology will quickly realize that this was not an easy feat!

It is not only technology that advances. Previous empirical gerontological research and theory, considered to be rock-solid in their era, continue to be modified, discarded or replaced by new findings and new paradigms. Models and theories continue to emerge that explain the current state of aging and old age much better than earlier frameworks still covered in many textbooks on aging and technology. It is little consolation that the aging process per se seems to be relatively invariant ("changing slowly," see preface in this volume by Neil Charness), because the heterogeneity of the aged, the aging, and the phenomenon of aging itself are tremendous.

Although the book is divided into five sections, they need not be read consecutively for understanding single chapters, and we have combined and sequenced them in such a way as to encourage the reader to build a well-organized cognitive or conceptual map of the contents of this book and the field of gerotechnology. After exploring the book, the astute reader may note alternative ways of organizing the chapters, but we believe that ours provides a parsimonious heuristic, and others may as well.

The title of Section A is "Basic Aspects of Gerotechnology." Here, our use of the term "basic" is to connote some fundamental aspects of the field that may or may not be familiar to the researcher, practitioner, or student reader from a variety of disciplines, but for which a basic understanding is necessary in order that technological innovations might have the greatest probability of successful application. For example, it is necessary to understand the underlying characteristics of the aging human in their social context (the biopsychosocial model) in order to best develop technological innovations. In addition, it is important to note that at the core of gerotechnology is the aim of "universal" accessibility.

In chapter 1, Rogers, Mayhorn, and Fisk provide an introduction to the issues and potential of gerotechnology by describing typical problems of older adults and technology in everyday life that can readily be translated into accessibility issues. For example, the trends should be (and generally are) that extra-individual factors become less important, because technology that fits individuals must be provided—the individual should not need to adapt to technology! On the other hand, it will not be possible in all instances to account for all idiosyncrasies of senior citizens. Hence, usability, training, and cognition aspects discussed in that chapter will continue to be part of gerotechnology, even after the (likely) advent of non-PC-based devices.

In that vein, Scialfa, Ho, and Laberge in chapter 2 and Mayhorn, Rogers, and Fisk in chapter 3 provide in-depth discussion of perceptual and cognitive aspects of aging that must be considered in gerotechnological innovations and interventions. One of the main conclusions we can draw here is the futility of constructing universal solutions—the multiplicity of biopsychosocial characteristics of human beings as well as the accumulation, combination, and potential interaction of such characteristics will stay with us forever, as far as we can imagine. Elder-prevalent deficits can be compensated for, or assisted by, present and future means, but at the time of this writing, Scialfa and colleagues view access to the world via technology as a burden to elders that is discordant with characteristics of the physical aging process. While their technical design specifications may become outdated as technologies advance, the principles of vision, hearing, and the tactile/haptic senses upon which the authors base their recommendations are likely to pass the test of time because of their implications for accessible design and usability standards.

Mayhorn, Rogers, and Fisk adopt an approach similar to Scialfa and colleagues by focusing on selected cognitive aging characteristics. Their examples, too, are illustrative for the reader in 2004 (although perhaps less so in 2014), and the evidence and principles they use as anchors for the design of technology will last until 2024 and beyond.

Assuming a social-science perspective on gerotechnology and various classical theories, as well as a theoretical theme particularly tied to technology, Mollenkopf, in chapter 4, furnishes broad-ranged analysis, and she obliquely criticizes the data-driven and immediate-troubleshooting-focused stance of the field. In employing ecological theory, she particularly succeeds in putting the role of the aging or aged individual into proper perspective: the "residual," "complicating factor," or "error" is not and does not rest with the human being—it is a function of the environment of which technology is a part. This position differs from "human factors" (or ergonomics), mentioned in several other chapters, where in a very technology-centered fashion the inherent assumption is that the human being constitutes the "disturbance." Access remains an issue. However, access and accessibility problems are inherent both in the description of socializational and socio-economic hindrances, as well as in the potential imbalance in person-environment fit that is an essential dynamic in ecological theories such as the competence model described in the chapters by Mollenkopf and Watzke in a later section.

Sections B and C cover areas that we consider to be the core activity fields of gerotechnology—computers and assistive devices. Here we had to compromise. Section B covers diverse aspects of computer usage by elders and their caregivers, and Section C discusses assistive technologies related to aging. While the distinction reflects currently separated activities, there is clear overlap in applications. Furthermore, there is no guarantee that computers will forever be the main device for communication and information acquisition, dissemination, and/or exchange, or for off-line applications. Microprocessor-controlled technology does not need to be confined by the limits of stationary or portable PCs. It is already possible to integrate most PC functions into smaller devices, such as wristwatch-type equipment, PDAs, or cell phones. The following example may not represent the most current technology in use, and it will be promptly superseded by newer, state-of-the-art technologies.

At one editor's university, multiple functions for cell phones and PDAs are available to and widely used by students, staff, and faculty using mostly wireless (infrared) transmission protocols, for example, use of the library, sundry payment systems on the whole continuum for the purchase of soft drinks at vending machines, parking cards, public transportation across the whole Seoul metropolitan area, and even credit card purchases. The devices are also used with automatic teller machines. They intertwine with Web-call services, and information about university-related issues, events, reminders, etc., all tailored to the individual's needs, and sent out as short text messages. Registration for and cancellation of classes, as well as management of grades are also at one's fingertips. On-campus phone calls are not charged, student attendance in classes can be electronically checked, and entrance to secured areas such as computer server rooms can be regulated. Apart from the school's own system, cell phones are also being connected to become traffic guidance systems for drivers, telling them in real-time where they are and which routes to use (and which to avoid); they can also be connected to live TV and video-on-demand services.

This example demonstrates the artificiality of the present distinction between PCs and other assistive devices. And although the applications above are focused on college students as end consumers, it is not difficult to imagine how such technology could be adapted to and modified for applied gerontological settings. This also illustrates the potential usage of a singular kind of multipurpose technology for different ages and aims.

In the first chapter of Section B, "Computers and Older Adults," Morrell, Mayhorn, and Echt summarize and analyze current trends of Internet usage by senior citizens, as well as understood, misunderstood, and other promoting and hindering factors, mostly from psychology. In terms of accessibility, the message conveyed is that there *are* barriers associated with aging, but that these can be removed or at least partially compensated for. Benbow concretely describes more barriers, as well as some of the ways to overcome them, in the following chapter, in particular with regard to evaluation of the quality of health information on the Internet. The salient accessibility issue at hand here is *not* that information is not accessible. On the contrary, it is the availability of *too much* information that prevents access to what is needed and useful. Smyth and Kwon discuss computer-mediated communication (CMC) with the focus on caregivers. It is particularly noteworthy that we are indeed dealing with communication modalities here that defy a certain degree of further optimization, e.g., the ways in which CMC is used will quite surely not be subject to sudden change as is the case with some other technological devices. Moreover, precisely the range of CMC options and the characteristics of different CMC modalities make some of them more accessible than other gerotechnological applications. Yet another aspect of accessibility has been presented by Burdick and others elsewhere (Burdick, 2003; Burdick & Michaels, 2003), namely encouragement of intergenerational relationships, i.e., the facilitation of communication by elders with other generations. Space limitations in this volume prohibited inclusion of an entire chapter on this topic, but it is worth mentioning here that this approach to the use of technology in our rapidly changing world holds much promise.

Section C has been titled "Assistive Technology, Home and Environment." While this important area has emerged from and still is very closely associated with the rehabilitation sciences and rehabilitation engineering, the distinction has become blurred over time and, as explained above, we predict that it will eventually become a less suitable criterion to categorize the field of gerotechnology in terms of PC and assistive technologies usage by elders—but at the time of this writing, this breakdown is still appropriate, because it reflects two different camps of mostly researchers and practitioners differing in professional background and activities with not yet much overlap.

For example, the anecdote of Hammel in the introductory chapter of Section C is a real eye-opener: Even with a relative in the family who has the highest expertise in assistive technology (AT) imaginable—*availability of* technology is not synonymous with *accessibility to* technology. The mere presence of devices is not enough. It takes human beings and, thus, the multidisciplinary efforts of technology-oriented and non-technology-oriented fields to ensure the effective and efficient use of AT and technology per se to meet unmet needs. Hammel describes these and similar changes in the AT field as, for instance, those affected by "universal design," which can be rephrased as "universal access" (although there are experts who would disagree—commonly accepted definitions of these and related terms do not exist). She discusses unresolved issues such as acceptance of AT and loss of privacy that are, like many other problems associated with gerotechnology and investigated in other chapters of this book, most likely to be grappled with for a very long time—if not always.

The monitoring of elders' behavior in their households as presented by Kutzik and Glascock does not seem to involve the pervasive accessibility perspective—at first sight. The authors describe a monitoring solution that may change with the kind of technology used over time, but both the distinctions they draw among presently available systems, and the components identified, are not that likely to change, e.g., the monitor itself (data collection), the processing module (data transformation and analysis), and the output (interface and data interpretation) with subsequent contingent actions taken. In terms of accessibility, we are dealing with a special instance of "technology as a primary means" to access information about oneself (or one's relative) in interaction with the environment by technical means under special circumstances, e.g., emergency situations, and/or if the older person is unable to access the information (because of loss of consciousness, panic, or lack of knowledge).

The chapter by Parker and Sabata complements Kutzik and Glascock and adds important insights by covering a broad field of safety technology (including issues related to crime and abuse) in a comprehensive senior-citizen residence typology for the purpose of discussing the diverse requirements to be met.

Tran offers insights into presently unique biomonitoring systems and provides an optimistic outlook regarding the potential of e-health or telemedical applications for the not-so-distant future, both at a full-fledged interventional level and at a level concentrating on preventive ends. Some technology described will remind the reader of aspects discussed by Kutzik and Glascock. Such common points emphasize the notion of shared underlying principles, which are in need of systematic investigation. An additional lesson to be learned is that it is not necessarily the highest-tech appliances that meet the needs of the elderly for independent living and well-being. Sometimes, a plain old phone will do.

Section D has been titled "Models, Prototypes, and Specific Applications of Gerotechnology." In this section, we included chapters that describe useful heuristic or procedural models of gerotechnology development—either from other fields of study (Ujimoto) or from within the field (Watzke; Dienel & Cameron)—which provide systems or systematic approaches for the development, testing, production and distribution of gerotechnological innovations. We also included a comprehensive chapter that underscores the importance of gerotechnology analysis in an important domain of function—driver safety (Rebok & Keyl).

Ujimoto approaches the topic from a long career in the application of human factors and ergonomics to airline performance and safety, viewing the gerotechnology field in a systemic fashion and using potentials to enhance or maintain elders' well-being as the cardinal yardstick. His analysis, which can be seen as an extension of the one provided by Mollenkopf in Section A, is reminiscent of cultural-anthropological and early 20th century sociological accounts. Ujimoto, too, is skeptical of the universal design idea ("one size fits all"). He also stresses what we see as another robustly time-insensitive aspect, namely the reduction of accident proneness by thorough analysis, inclusion of (so-called) redundant systems, effective communication structures, and the like. Experiences in the aviation industry have clear relevance to various issues of gerotechnology—as Ujimoto directly notes with regard to health care and older adults, but with another logical relationship to elder driver safety.

The assessment of driving ability, the validity of the instruments, and the consequences for modeling technology and/or inducing behavioral change in elderly individuals are described by Rebok and Keyl. As western populations age rapidly, particularly in the United States where automobiles (particularly SUVs) are the main mode of transportation (more ubiquitous than computers at this juncture in time), the clash of population aging with the potential for car crashes provides a fertile area of investigation for gerotechnologists.

Watzke's chapter on the Dr. Tong Louie Living Laboratory in Vancouver presents a sample case for the organization and logistics involved in developing and maintaining an optimized gerotechnology laboratory. Although there are several idiosyncrasies that needed to be accounted for to get and keep the lab up and running, the basic steps involved, as well as the ideas and principles related to staffing, funding, or kinds of research are readily generalizable across place and time, and serve as useful instruction for those wishing to develop their own centers. The chapter also presents a vivid account of seemingly trite, but actually not that trivial, practical arrangements for (1) the much-called-for but not-much-implemented multidisciplinary and/or interdisciplinary cooperation in the field of applied gerontology, and (2) bridging the gap between research and practice in the form of actual mass production and the cultivation of marketability (so-called "translational research").

Dienel and Cameron discuss elderly consumer participation in AT development. While their particular approach is not yet mainstream, it is generally a *sine qua non* to involve the users-to-be in product development—now as well as in the future. We may be able to think of consumer behavior as calculable, e.g., as an objective for simulation. Indeed, in some instances, it is not only unnecessary, but mandatory to simulate instead of to test technology with human subjects, for instance in vehicle crash tests. However, for now and for the foreseeable future, participatory design is a mandate that is all too often neglected.

In the final section, entitled "Cautions, Integration, and Synthesis," we have included a provocative chapter urging caution, and an integrative and comprehensive epilogue. These chapters may give a new perspective or context to ideas and innovations explored earlier in the text.

Students of business are now quite familiar with the SWOT model—the need to evaluate the strengths, weaknesses, opportunities, and threats of any new action, development, or product. While the majority of this book has focused primarily upon the incredible strengths and opportunities provided by the application of technology to the needs and wants of older adults, it is necessary to carefully consider the threats or perils. Certainly Ujimoto described some significant risks if technology isn't carefully applied in the health care setting. Many other chapters also noted the downside of inappropriately designed technology. (We are reminded of research by Wendy Rogers, alluded to in chapter

1, about blood glucose meters purportedly as "easy as 1– 2– 3" actually involving over 30 discrete steps and resulting in clinically significant mistakes in over 50% of study subjects). But, Lesnoff-Caravaglia faces us squarely with significant concerns about gerotechnology. If you didn't know her as one of the pioneers in the field of gerotechnology, you might believe Dr. Lesnoff-Caravaglia to be a Luddite. Nothing could be further from the truth. But, in this chapter, she goes beyond the usual ethical discussion. Here she explores the hazard of neglecting the individual in this complex, aging world. While the advantages brought about by new technologies cannot be denied, they have become both causes of and aggravating factors for ethical dangers at present, in the near future, and in a very distant future when technology really may be virtually timeless and when this book will indeed be only of historical value and accessibility issues an anachronism.

The book ends with an Epilogue by Dr. James Fozard, another pioneer in gerotechnology/gerontechnology. From his unique vantage point, Dr. Fozard discusses how this field of study has developed over nearly a half century. He notes that his introduction to the concept of human factors (ergonomics) in 1956 referred to it as "engineering for human use," and that the term "had nothing to do with aging." Fozard suggest that both the study of aging and human factors (ergonomics) have benefited greatly by having *much* to do with one another in the ensuing years.

In sum, we believe that this is a first-rate collection of ideas from a variety of leaders in this field and we believe that it makes a substantial and substantive contribution to the body of literature on technology and aging. We are therefore grateful to all of our authors and readers.

—Sunkyo Kwon and
David C. Burdick
January 2004

REFERENCES

Burdick, D. C. (2003, November). The changing world of intergenerational relations: Computers bridge generation gap, enhance well-being for young and old. Symposium presented at the 56th Annual Scientific Meeting of the Gerontological Society of America, San Diego, California.

Burdick, D. C., & Michaels, M. (2003). *The generation gap and computer technology: How computers and the Internet can bring generations together.* Unpublished manuscript.

Preface

We are in the midst of two striking trends: widespread population aging and rapid diffusion of technology. Both phenomena are very new in human history. As an example, life expectancy in 1900 in the U.S. was about 50 years. Today it is approaching 80 years. In terms of technology diffusion, it is worth noting that the patent for a facsimile (fax) machine was granted in 1843, but it took about 150 years before it was widely adopted. Even the indispensable telephone (patented in 1876) took about 40–50 years to become widely distributed in the U.S. The pace has quickened in recent times, with perhaps about 20–30 years before the consumer microwave oven (produced in 1967 by Amana in the U.S.) became widespread. It took only about 10 years for 50% of U.S. households to acquire access to the World Wide Web (protocol defined in 1989 and the first browser developed in 1992).

Advances in both these areas are in part a by-product of population-level wealth accumulation and its reciprocal relation to knowledge, particularly scientific knowledge. That is, societies that have sufficient resources to safeguard the basic needs of their populations can afford to invest in the pursuit of knowledge, and that pursuit usually leads to high returns on investment in the form of better knowledge and greater resource generation. This virtuous circle promises to accelerate the two trends of longevity and technology diffusion.

Population aging has good and bad features. A popular joke describes a birthday party where the centenarian was asked how it felt to be 100 years old. The person replied: "Not bad, when you consider the alternative." More life is better than less life most of the time. However, old age, particularly advanced old age, (what Baltes has termed the fourth age) is usually a time of diminished abilities, diminished health, and diminished financial and social resources. Modern technology has the potential to enhance human health, abilities, and relationships. A good example is how modern communication technologies (postal services, telegraph, telephone, e-mail) have made it possible to carry on long-distance relationships successfully.

We face an interesting set of challenges in trying to meld these two trends. Technology, when designed with older users in mind, can contribute to greater productivity, comfort, and safety for older adults. However, technology comes with a price tag, and often a high one when products are first introduced. If you examine the studies of computer diffusion in the U.S., it is clear that early on, when computer prices were high, those who adopted them were in the upper income levels. As prices came down, economic status was less of a barrier to adoption. Old age is usually a time of waning resources. Retirement from paid work, a very new phenomenon in human history, typically begins around age 62–65 in the U.S., and immediately diminishes spending power. Very old age cohorts are populated today mainly by women who, at this time in history, have not accumulated a great deal of wealth during their working years (compared with men). Thus, the ability to pay for technological advancements, that for instance might combat or ameliorate the effects of chronic diseases, declines with increasing age. Providing the fruits of technological advances to those with limited spending power is a persistent challenge for all societies.

This volume aims to address both specific and general issues in the new field of gerontechnology/gerotechnology. Section A addresses issues in person-environment fit for technology, and deals with age-related changes in capabilities, accessibility to and design for technology, as well as cultural constraints in its adoption and use. Section B focuses on arguably the most important and most powerful artifact of the past century, the digital computer and the Internet, the electronic network that increasingly links us to other people, goods, and services. Section C addresses the practical issue of how to apply technology to assist people in overcoming the types of impairments that tend to increase exponentially as people pass their middle adult years. Section D looks at broad areas, models, or prototypes for technology development and the application of technology to everyday life, including the increasingly important domains of health care and driver safety. Section E provides ethical cautions and additional integration and synthesis of materials covered earlier in the book. The reader will find these chapters to be informative, engaging, and most important of all, thought provoking.

In contrast to technology that is changing rapidly over time, aging people, fortunately, change slowly. Except for the case of acute onset of health problems, and as a result of this slow rate of change, people usually have time to adapt to their waning capabilities. Technology, when properly designed, deployed, and supported, promises to be an important ally to all those who now and in the future must adapt to their aging bodies and minds. This volume provides a very informative and broad-ranging examination of the current state of technology and its role in our increasingly prevalent process of adaptation to aging.

Neil Charness, PhD
Professor of Psychology and Research Associate
Pepper Institute on Aging and Public Policy
Florida State University
Tallahassee, Florida

Acknowledgments

The editors wish to thank several individuals and organizations without whose assistance this manuscript would not have been produced. First, we thank all of our authors for their good work, goodwill, and patience in the lengthy process of bringing this work to press. In particular, Neil Charness and Jim Fozard provided valuable insights and moral support during the editing process. We also wish to acknowledge the assistance and participation of many individuals from the Formal Interest Group on Technology and Aging of the Gerontological Society of America (GSA-TAG). Several of GSA-TAG's members as well as its current convener, Mary Parker, are authors in this volume. It has been a pleasure working with Springer Publishing and its representatives. We are particularly grateful to Shoshana Bauminger, Assistant Editor, Sheri W. Sussman, Editorial Director, and Jeanne Libby, Assistant Production Manager, for their assistance and guidance. David Burdick's work was partially supported by The Richard Stockton College of New Jersey through a one-semester sabbatical, travel support for several conferences, and secretarial assistance in the Division of Social and Behavioral Sciences. Special thanks go to Patricia Pruitt for her assistance with proofreading. Finally, both editors wish to express our deep gratitude to our families and extended professional families.

Section A

Basic Aspects of
Gerotechnology

1

Technology in Everyday Life for Older Adults

Wendy A. Rogers,
Christopher B. Mayhorn,
and Arthur D. Fisk

Jerry is retired and lives at home with his wife Carol. When Jerry gets up in the morning he uses the electric coffee maker to make his coffee and the microwave oven to heat his oatmeal. After breakfast he goes to the computer to check for e-mail from his children. He has received several messages, some with attachments and pictures that he prints out for Carol to read later. He decides to go out for a ride—he must first set the house alarm, and then turn off the car alarm so he does not wake all the neighbors. Entering the car he programs his global positioning system (GPS) to obtain directions to the new golf store the next town over. At the golf store he purchases a new putter—using the store's self-checkout system. Jerry must scan his putter and then use the credit card reader to pay for his purchase. On the way home, he stops at the library to get a book he has wanted to read. He first looks up the proper spelling for the author's name as he had noted it in his personal digital assistant. He then uses the online card catalog to find the location of the book in the library stacks. Back at home, he turns off the house alarm and checks his answering machine for messages. His physician has left an automated message reminding him of his appointment the following afternoon. Deciding to relax for a while, Jerry inserts the digital videodisk (DVD) that came with his new putter into the DVD player. He then remembers he must check his blood glucose before lunch, so he uses his electronic blood glucose meter to assess his current level so he can adjust his medication and decide what to have for lunch.

This vignette illustrates current technology available in the life of older adults. Individuals may interact with a wide variety of interfaces, displays, input and output devices, all before lunch! Technology has the potential to make life easier, to support communication with family and friends, to assist with health care, and to enable individuals to remain safe and functionally independent in their own homes. However, Jerry may be somewhat of a trendsetter and not all older adults are technology-savvy with access to all of the latest, greatest gadgets and gizmos. Moreover, many devices and systems are difficult to use, they do not always seem to work properly, or they are so complex as to seem beyond one's capabilities.

The focus of this chapter is technology in the lives of older adults. We will discuss the validity of myths about older adults' attitudes and willingness to use new technologies. We will then describe the design and training factors that may impede the use of technology by older adults. We will conclude the chapter with a discussion of the potential for future technology and the barriers that must be understood and overcome to meet this potential.

MYTHOLOGY OF OLDER ADULTS AND TECHNOLOGY USE

"Older adults prefer to do things the old-fashioned way." "You can't teach an old dog new tricks." "New technologies are for the young." While it is true that older adults are slower to adopt many new technologies, and typically require more training to learn to use them, these myths about older adults and new technologies are greatly overstated (see also Morrell, Mayhorn, & Echt, this volume).

Here are some of the facts about use of technology by older adults:

1. 40% of people over age 65 use computers (U.S. Department of Commerce, 2002)
2. 35% of people over age 65 access the Internet (U.S. Department of Commerce)
3. 90% of older adults own a microwave oven, 80% own videocassette recorders, and 60% own cordless phones and answering machines (Adler, 1996)

While these statistics reflect the willingness of only American older adults to adopt new technology, it is important to realize that older adults in nations around the world are making similar decisions. The National Aging Information Center (2002) recently reported several statistics that highlight the growth of technology usage by older adults in several countries. For instance, Australian seniors are the largest growing segment of online banking service users, totaling over 775,000. The number of senior Internet users in the United Kingdom recently surpassed 2 million, accounting for approximately 13% of that nation's online population. Sweden and Denmark, however, boast the highest percentage of senior Internet users in Europe with 17% and 16% percent of their respective national Internet user populations. The percentage of Canadian seniors using the Internet and computers has also steadily increased over the last decade (National Advisory Council on Aging, 2001).

These data clearly indicate that many older adults in developed nations have daily interactions with technology. In fact, the rate of technology development in society is making it difficult for them to avoid it. Most businesses today do not have a person answering the telephone; instead they have an automated telephone menu. The library has an online search system rather than a card catalog. At the grocery store you are expected to scan your own credit card, and in some stores scan your own groceries.

Asking why some older adults do not use new technologies is a relevant question. However, it must be accompanied by questions about why older adults encounter difficulties using technologies, why they have difficulty learning new systems, and how the development of future technologies should be directed to meet the needs of older adults.

WHAT REALLY IMPEDES USE OF TECHNOLOGY BY OLDER ADULTS?

A valuable starting point for understanding the difficulties older adults encounter when using technologies is to ask them. In a focus group study, Rogers, Meyer, Walker, and Fisk (1998) interviewed groups of older adults between the ages of 65 and 80 and asked them about frustrations and difficulties they encounter when carrying out their normal daily activities. Although the group discussions were not specifically focused on technology, one interesting finding was the variety of technologies encountered by individuals in their everyday lives. Most germane to the present discussion, however, were the frustrations that seemed to accompany use of technology. Table 1.1 contains some quotes from participants in this study.

To determine the source of the difficulties that older adults were experiencing, Rogers, Meyer, Walker, and Fisk (1998) coded each difficulty reported by their older adult participants (technology-related and otherwise). Each problem was classified according to whether it was

TABLE 1.1 Older Adults' Frustrations with Technologies Indicate Usability Problems

Technology	Quote from Older Adult
Videocassette Recorder	I cannot do that VCR. I can't program that and I have read those directions over and over.
Entertainment Center	My entertainment center . . . somebody told me I could get a all-around remote for it and, I got the remote and I got mad 'cause I couldn't hook it up, so . . . real disgusted, threw it across the room.
Photocopier	Some of these new copy machines, those massive things . . . some of these things you've got now they throw them out and staple 'em . . . But I ain't got brains enough to learn to use 'em.
Camera	Well, I have a camera that I can't operate. I can get the film in there and I can never get it out. I always have to take it to the photo place and say, "please take this film out."
Fax Machine	I would like to fax a letter. I needed to get a letter in a hurry, and I had access to the machine, but I didn't know how to do it. It made me mad.
In-vehicle Technology	We recently had a rental car . . . that array of buttons in the front of you, you know it just unnerves you . . . it did for me . . . I never learned what all the buttons did in the two weeks we had the car.
Online Library Catalog	Well I'm frustrated in the library . . . When they sit you down in front of a computer and they tell you to look it up here. I have to have somebody tell me where to put my fingers.
Electric Mixer	I bought a new mixer and God knows I haven't learned how to use it yet, it's a shame, a new mixer . . . but it's these, ah, modern things you just don't hardly know how to use them.
Word Processor	Word processor! I had to learn the computer when I was fifty years old. It was rough. I remember telling my boss you can teach old dog new tricks, but it's awfully hard on that old dog.

Note. These quotes are from the focus groups conducted by Rogers, Meyer, Walker, and Fisk (1998).

potentially remediable through some human factors intervention such as improved training or instruction, redesign of the system or the environment, a combination of training and redesign, or neither training nor design could solve the problem. Forty-seven percent of the problems fell into the latter category—that is, older adults reported health problems or medical problems that were not likely to be remedied by any human factors intervention. However, the remaining 53% of the problems could potentially be solved by improvements in design, training, or a combination of the two. Rogers and colleagues did not mean to imply that the solutions were readily available—only that they were potentially available. But for the solutions to be realized we must understand the specific design factors and training issues that may influence older adults' interactions with technology. Also, research must ultimately be translated into practice (see Fisk, Rogers, Charness, Czaja, & Sharit, 2004).

DESIGN FACTORS

Design issues can impede use of everyday products. Hancock, Fisk, and Rogers (2001) queried adults about their experiences with various common household products. As shown in Table 1.2, participants of all ages reported usability problems with these familiar products. User difficulties resulted from text that was difficult to understand, symbols that could not be interpreted, perceptual difficulties seeing the print or what was to be manipulated, and motor difficulties using the product. Memory difficulties were also reported, but less frequently for the older adults. Perhaps the older adults did not remember having memory problems (an ironic consequence of declining memory) or had developed compensatory strategies so that they no longer experienced memory difficulties when using common household products.

While Hancock and colleagues' (2001) survey did not focus on technology per se, the reported usability difficulties are indicative of the types of problems that people of all ages encounter when interacting with artifacts. These data also provide a framework for understanding design characteristics of technologies that affect usability, namely comprehension factors related to text and symbols (or icons), perceptual or motor issues, and cognitive factors such as memory. Designers must understand the perceptual, motor control, and cognitive capabilities of users, and in particular how such abilities change as a function of age. Other chapters in this volume address these issues in more depth (Mayhorn, Rogers, & Fisk; Scialfa, Ho, & LaBerge).

TABLE 1.2 Percentage of Participants Reporting Usability Problems and Types of Problems

	Young (18–35)	Middle-Aged (36–54)	Young-Old (55–64)	Old (65–91)
Category of Product				
Healthcare Product	39	41	40	44
Over-the-counter Medication	53	57	58	50
Cleaner	49	50	50	48
Toiletry	36	44	44	43
Category of Usability Problem (for those reporting difficulties)				
Text Comprehension	27	32	30	26
Symbol Comprehension	12	22	25	23
Perceptual Difficulties	26	57	55	51
Memory Difficulties	66	51	46	48
Motor Difficulties	80	80	80	94

Note. These data are from the product usage survey conducted by Hancock, Fisk, and Rogers (2001).

TRAINING ISSUES

As noted above, human factors interventions that support the activities of older adults include the development of instruction and training. Although system design can almost always be improved, even the best-designed system will likely require some training for novice users (consider automobiles and computers). Furthermore, instruction or training is often required for experienced users to be able to use all of the functionality available in the system (consider a personal digital assistant or a cellular telephone). The aging process may also result in the need for age-specific instructional design that enables older individuals to safely and effectively interact with technologies (see the chapters in this volume by Benbow and by Morrell, Mayhorn, & Echt). Technology itself may yield improvements in training design such as using a simulator for driver retraining as described in this volume by Rebok and Keyl.

Older adults exhibit declines in abilities shown to be important for learning and skill acquisition. Such abilities include fluid intelligence, working memory, perceptual speed, and spatial ability (Rogers, Hertzog, & Fisk, 2000). Older adults learn new skills; yet, proper instructional design that capitalizes on intact abilities and compensates for declining abilities holds much promise for proficient novice level performance, substantive proficiency gains with training (Jamieson & Rogers, 2000; Mead & Fisk, 1998; Rogers, Fisk, Mead, Walker, & Cabrera, 1996), and retention of proficient levels of system usage (Fisk, Hertzog, Lee, Rogers, & Anderson-Garlach, 1994). Proper training coupled with adequate system design can lead to dramatic increases in system usage accuracy for older adults (see Rogers, Fisk, Mead, Walker, & Cabrera, 1996; Sharit, Czaja, Nair, & Lee, 2003). Moreover, older adults have expressed a desire to receive training even for technologies such as automated teller machines that are presumed to be usable by virtually anyone with no experience needed (Rogers, Cabrera, Walker, Gilbert, & Fisk, 1996) or an online library catalog (Rousseau, Jamieson, Rogers, Mead, & Sit, 1998).

RECOGNITION OF POTENTIAL BENEFITS IS IMPORTANT

Systems must be well designed and proper training must be provided. Does that guarantee that older adults will adopt new technologies to perform daily tasks? Not necessarily—adoption of new technologies is influenced by several factors such as the relative advantage of the technology (in comparison with previous methods of accomplishing the activity) and the degree to which the innovation is compatible with one's values, experiences, and needs (Rogers, 1995). Of course, accessibility also contributes to adoption, as does the organizational culture of the climate in which the technology is introduced (Ujimoto, this volume), and other macro-level issues such as changing social and technical environments (Mollenkopf, this volume).

Factors that influence adoption of new communication technologies were investigated by Melenhorst, Rogers, and Bouwhuis (2003) (see also Melenhorst, 2002; Melenhorst, Rogers, & Caylor, 2001). In a focus group study, older adults were asked how they would decide what communication method would be best suited for a particular communication goal such as sharing good news or making an appointment. Internet users and nonusers were queried about their preference to use the telephone, a face-to-face visit, a letter, or the Internet. Of particular interest was the reasoning the participants used—why they selected a particular method of communication. The results revealed that older adults made their decisions primarily on the basis of the perceived benefits (or lack thereof) of the particular communication method afforded by the technology. These data indicated that the decision process seemed to rely mostly on whether the method suited their needs (i.e., was fast enough or personal enough or easy enough). Contrary to myths about use of technology by older adults, their decisions were not primarily based on issues such as whether the method was too difficult, too financially costly, or too time-intensive to learn. These data support the notion that technology will be adopted by individuals when its benefits are clear to them and meet their needs. Older adults seem willing to invest the time, resources, and money necessary to learn new technologies, if such benefits are clear.

The Melenhorst, Rogers and Bouwhuis (2003) data were collected in both the United States and The Netherlands and the pattern of results was strikingly similar across the two nations. However, there is some limited evidence that adoption of new technologies in developing countries may be influenced by different factors such as social pressure (Anandarajan, Igbaria, & Anakwe, 2000), which did not arises as an important factor in the Melenhorst, Rogers and Bouwhuis study.

MEETING THE POTENTIAL FOR FUTURE TECHNOLOGIES

An innovative research program at the Georgia Institute of Technology (Georgia Tech) is focused on developing computer technology to support the independence and quality of life of older adults by enabling them to remain in their own homes. This Aware Home Research Initiative consists of an interdisciplinary team of computer scientists, engineers, and psychologists (www.cc.gatech.edu/fce/ahri/index.html). Their research and development activities are carried out in a residential laboratory (i.e., a high-tech home) on the Georgia Tech campus. (For additional details about Aware Home research efforts, see Essa, 2000; Kidd, Orr, Abowd, Atkeson, Essa, et al., 1999; Mynatt, Essa, & Rogers, 2000; Mynatt & Rogers, 2002.)

The Aware Home Research Initiative is certainly not the only effort to develop computing technology to support elders in their home environment. Other examples are discussed in this volume by Hammel; Kutzik and Glascock; Parker and Sabata; and Tran. Descriptions of other worldwide efforts of "smart" homes, or domotics, are available online at www.smart-homes.nl;www.sentha.tu-berlin.de/www.stakes.fi/cost219/smarthousing.htm; www.gdewsbury.ukideas.com; and www.cc.gatech.edu/fce/ahri/index.html (for a recent review see van Berlo, 2002). In brief, existing efforts have focused on areas of safety (fire, smoke, intrusion), comfort (heat, lights, shades), communication (telephones, videophones, teleshopping, telehealth, telework), entertainment (device control, VCR programming), and remote management. In fact, a smart home is defined as "a home or working environment, which includes the technology to allow for devices and systems to be controlled automatically" (van Berlo, 1999, p. 6).

The Aware Home Research Initiative is meant to go beyond the "control" of home systems. The computing applications are intended to augment the activities of the people living in the home—supporting their activities, providing interactive information to the home dwellers and selected individuals outside of the home, and enabling the development of predictive models of changes in capabilities based on trending information.

Successful independent living requires older adults to be capable of performing basic Activities of Daily Living (ADLs) such as bathing, toileting, and eating, as well as more instrumental activities of daily living (IADLs) such as managing a medication regimen, maintaining the household, and preparing nutritious meals (Lawton, 1990). Existence as an independently living, active older adult may also require willingness to accept new challenges and to engage in lifelong learning, referred to as enhanced activities of daily living (EADLs) (Rogers, Meyer, Walker, & Fisk, 1998). All of the activities can potentially be aided by augmented environments, for example ADL supports during bathing such as temperature regulation and monitoring the vital signs of the bather for signs of problems; IADL supports such as external cues to enhance medication-taking behavior, nutritional information, and support for meal-preparation; and EADL supports that facilitate social communication and enhance leisure activities.

BARRIERS TO BE UNDERSTOOD AND OVERCOME

Future research in advanced computing technologies must explore how computers can enhance day-to-day activities. The computer should not be thought of as a tool to be picked up, used, and then set aside—it can be a constant partner in daily activities. This is the concept of ubiquitous computing where the computer is embedded everywhere, seamlessly integrated into one's everyday activities (Weiser, 1991). The computer could notice when you are interrupted and help you regain your task. It could monitor your environment, and inform you of useful information. It could help you schedule your day to coordinate virtual visits from health care personnel and actual visits from family and friends.

An important challenge is to design interfaces that reflect and support the ongoing activity of daily life but are not inappropriately intrusive. Some of the issues are specific to the aging individual, such as what activities need to be supported, how the level of support should change to accommodate the changing needs of the individual, and how to develop interfaces that will be usable by older persons and their family members. Other issues are more general to the nature of home-based ubiquitous computing such as technical, social, and pragmatic issues (Edwards & Grinter, 2001). Methods for development and testing of prototype systems are described in this volume by Watzke, and by Dienel, Peine, and Cameron.

To design effective systems and training programs in support of age-related performance capabilities, we must answer fundamental questions concerning aging and complex task performance. This requires a clear understanding of the needs and priorities of older adults relative to health, well being, and safety, as well as their view of technology solutions. For example, knowing that older adults have working memory deficits and attention problems, or that they process information more slowly than young adults, is necessary but not sufficient for motivating solutions to design-related problems. An understanding of age-related changes in cognition is essential in establishing design principles for the application of new technology. In addition, researchers need to better understand issues of privacy, acceptance, and trust as these issues relate to the development and use of technology in the homes of older adults. These factors are discussed below and other broad issues of ethics in technology and aging are described by Lesnoff-Caravaglia elsewhere in this volume.

PRIVACY

The presence of aware services in the home raises the issue of privacy. How much information is collected about the occupant and who is privy to that information? For example, in the design of monitoring systems, the individual who is being monitored should determine the type of information to be transmitted as well as the people with whom the information will be shared (Mynatt & Rogers, 2002). A related issue is security of collected, but not transmitted, information (see also Kutzik & Glascock, this volume). For example, raw video signals could be used by a service to determine and share changes in an occupant's gait following hip surgery. The raw video must be securely stored and later deleted to prevent unwanted disclosure.

Researchers must develop the scientific construct of privacy to understand how privacy concerns may change across contexts, individuals, and cultures. For example, in a non emergency situation, a person may be unwilling to relinquish any privacy, whereas in a life-threatening situation privacy may be of less concern. Privacy is really a multidimensional construct that is not yet well understood. Privacy concerns may be related to knowing when and what type of information is being collected, determining who has access to such information, and whether information can be subsequently linked to a particular person (Friedman & Kahn, 2003).

ACCEPTABILITY

Within home environments, a strategy for increasing acceptance of ubiquitous computing may be to introduce it gradually to older adults who are still high functioning (e.g., in their 50s and 60s) and to increase the supports provided by the technologies as motor control, perceptual, and cognitive abilities decline (e.g., in their 70s and 80s). An important research question is to determine how to identify these transition points—such decisions could be based on trending data from computational perception applications. Newell and his colleagues have discussed designing for "dynamic diversity" whereby designers recognize that systems must consider the diversity of capabilities within an individual at different points of time, not only as the person ages, but also when the person is operating in a stressful or time-pressured situation (e.g., Newell, Carmichael, Gregor, & Alm, 2003). Designing for such dynamic diversity should yield systems that adapt to the user's changing capabilities and such systems may be more acceptable because they neither underestimate nor overcompensate for the user's capabilities at a given point in time.

TRUST IN AUTOMATION

If technology is to be developed to support the independence of older adults in their homes, the technology must, of course, be reliable. Perhaps equally important, however, the person must be willing to rely on the technology. User decisions to rely on automated devices depend on their trust in the automation and self-confidence in their ability to control the system. Trust is dependent on current and prior levels of system performance, the presence of faults, and prior levels of trust. Bisanz and Seong (2001) proposed a multidimensional taxonomy of factors that affect trust in automated systems; however, their work focused on younger adults and little work has been conducted to date on the variables that influence trust in automated systems for older adults. Moreover, the degree to which one's confidence in the ability to control the system may prove particularly important for older adults with less technology experience.

CONCLUSIONS

Older adults are willing to use new technologies, contrary to some stereotyped views. Older adults are more accepting if they are provided with adequate training (Rogers, Fisk, Mead, Walker, & Cabrera, 1996) and if the benefits of the technology are clear to them (Melenhorst, Rogers, & Bouwhuis, 2003). Moreover, field trials of intelligent home monitoring systems have been implemented successfully with adults age 60–85 (e.g., Sixsmith, 2000).

The integration of computer technology with traditional assistive technologies and environmental modifications, can lead to interventions that will promote successful aging by enhancing the health, safety, independence, active engagement, and quality of life of older adults. We must follow human factors principles of understanding the needs of the user population, designing systems with their capabilities and limitations in mind, and providing appropriate training, instruction, and help systems to support performance (Rogers & Fisk, 2000). According to Pew, the human factors profession must serve as "the gatekeepers to ensure that the technological capabilities that are thrust on us will be manageable and responsive to human requirements . . . we have the opportunity to design the interfaces that translate that technology into tools and products that are useful, usable, meaningful, assessable, rewarding, and fun" (Pew, 2003, p. 15). The challenge that accompanies this opportunity is to provide designers with fundamental knowledge about older adults' characteristics, capabilities, concerns, competencies, and cares.

ACKNOWLEDGMENTS

Wendy A. Rogers is Professor and Associate Chair, School of Psychology, Georgia Institute of Technology. Christopher B. Mayhorn is Assistant Professor, Ergonomics & Experimental Psychology, North Carolina State University. Arthur D. Fisk is Professor, School of Psychology and Coordinator, Engineering Psychology, Georgia Institute of Technology.

The first and third authors were supported in part by a grant from the National Institutes of Health (National Institute on Aging) Grant P01 AG17211 under the auspices of the Center for Research and Education on Aging and Technology Enhancement (CREATE); Award 0121661 "The Aware Home: Sustaining the Quality of Life for an Aging Population" from the National Science Foundation; and the Aware Home Research Initiative industrial partners.

Correspondence concerning this chapter should be addressed to Wendy A. Rogers, School of Psychology, Georgia Institute of Technology, Atlanta, Georgia, 30332-0170. Electronic mail: wr43@mail.gatech.edu. Phone: 404-894-6775.

REFERENCES

Adler, R. P. (1996). Older adults and computers: Report of a national survey. *Technical Report for SeniorNet.*

Anandarajan, M., Igbaria, M., & Anakwe, U. P. (2000). Technology acceptance in the banking industry: A perspective from a less developed country. *Information Technology & People, 13,* 298–312.

Bisantz, A. M., & Seong, Y. (2001). Assessment of operator trust in and utilization of automated decision-aids under different framing conditions. *International Journal of Industrial Ergonomics, 28,* 85–97.

Edwards, W. K., & Grinter, R. E. (2001). At home with ubiquitous computing: Seven challenges. In G. D. Abowd, B. Brumitt, & S. A. N. Shafer (Eds.) *Ubicomp 2001, LNCS 2201.* Berlin: Springer-Verlag.

Essa, I. (2000). Ubiquitous Sensing for Smart and Aware Environments. In *IEEE Personal Communications, Special Issue on Networking the Physical World.*

Fisk, A. D., Hertzog, C., Lee, M. D., Rogers, W. A., & Anderson-Garlach, M. (1994). Long-term retention of skilled visual search: Do young adults retain more than old adults? *Psychology and Aging, 9,* 206–215.

Fisk, A. D., Rogers, W. A., Charness, N., Czaja, S. J., & Sharit, J. (2004). *Designing for older adults: Principles and creative human factors approaches.* London: Taylor and Francis.

Friedman, B., & Kahn, P. H. (2003). Human values, ethics, and design. In J. A. Jacko & A. Sears (Eds.), *The human-computer interaction handbook: Fundamentals, evolving technologies, and emerging applications.* Mahwah, NJ: Erlbaum.

Hancock, H. E., Fisk, A. D., & Rogers, W. A. (2001). Everyday products: Easy to use . . . or not? *Ergonomics in Design, 9,* 12–18.

Jamieson, B. A., & Rogers, W. A. (2000). Age-related effects of blocked and random practice schedules on learning a new technology. *Journals of Gerontology: Psychological Sciences, 55B,* P343—P353.

Kidd, C. D., Orr, R. J., Abowd, G. D., Atkeson, C. G., Essa, I. A., MacIntyre, B., et al. (1999). The Aware Home: A Living Laboratory for Ubiquitous Computing Research. Proceedings of the Second International Workshop on Cooperative Buildings, CoBuild'99.

Lawton, M. P. (1990). Aging and performance on home tasks. *Human Factors, 32,* 527–536.

Mead, S. E., & Fisk, A. D. (1998). Measuring skill acquisition and retention with an ATM simulator: The need for age-specific training. *Human Factors, 40,* 516–523.

Melenhorst, A. S. (2002). *Adopting communication technology in later life: The decisive role of benefits.* Eindhoven, The Netherlands: Technical University of Eindhoven.

Melenhorst, A. S., Rogers, W. A., & Bouwhuis, D. (2003). Unpublished manuscript.

Melenhorst, A. S., Rogers, W. A., & Caylor, E. C. (2001). The use of communication technologies by older adults: Exploring the benefits from the user's perspective. Proceedings of the Human Factors and Ergonomics Society 46th Annual Meeting. Santa Monica, California.

Mynatt, E. D., Essa, I., & Rogers, W. A. (2000). Increasing the Opportunities for Aging in Place. ACM Proceedings of the 2000 Conference on Universal Usability.

Mynatt, E. D., & Rogers, W. A. (2002). Developing technology to support the functional independence of older adults. *Ageing International, 27,* 24–41.

National Advisory Council on Aging (2001). *Seniors and technology.* Ottawa, Ontario: Canadian Public Works Printing Office.

National Aging Information Center (2002). Available at: www.aoa.gov

Newell, A. F., Carmichael, A., Gregor, P., & Alm, N. (2003). Information technology for cognitive support. In J. A. Jacko & A. Sears (Eds.), *The human-computer interaction handbook: Fundamentals, evolving technologies, and emerging applications.* Mahwah, NJ: Erlbaum.

Pew, R. W. (2003). Evolution of human-computer interaction: From memex to Bluetooth and beyond. In J. A. Jacko & A. Sears (Eds.), *The human-computer interaction handbook: Fundamentals, evolving technologies, and emerging applications.* Mahwah, NJ: Erlbaum.

Rogers, E. M. (1995). *Diffusion of innovations* (4th ed.). New York: The Free Press.

Rogers, W. A., Cabrera, E. F., Walker, N., Gilbert, D. K., & Fisk, A. D. (1996). A survey of automatic teller machine usage across the adult lifespan. *Human Factors, 38*, 156–166.

Rogers, W. A., & Fisk, A. D. (2000). Human factors, applied cognition, and aging. In F. I. M. Craik & T. A. Salthouse (Eds.), *The handbook of aging and cognition* (2nd ed.). Mahwah, NJ: Erlbaum.

Rogers, W. A., Fisk, A. D., Mead, S. E., Walker, N., & Cabrera, E. F. (1996). Training older adults to use automatic teller machines. *Human Factors, 38*, 425–433.

Rogers, W. A., Hertzog, C., & Fisk, A. D. (2000). Age-related differences in associative learning: An individual differences analysis of ability and strategy influences. *Journal of Experimental Psychology: Learning, Memory, and Cognition, 26*, 359–394.

Rogers, W. A., Meyer, B., Walker, N., & Fisk, A. D. (1998). Functional limitations to daily living tasks in the aged: A focus group analysis. *Human Factors, 40*, 111–125.

Rousseau, G. K., Jamieson, B. A., Rogers, W. A., Mead, S. E., & Sit, R. A. (1998). Assessing the usability of on-line library systems. *Behaviour and Information Technology, 17*, 274–281.

Sharit, J., Czaja, S. J., Nair, S., & Lee, C. C. (2003). Effects of age, speech rate, and environmental support in using telephone voice menu systems. *Human Factors, 45*, 234–252.

Sixsmith, A. J. (2000). An evaluation of an intelligent home monitoring system. *Journal of Telemedicine and Telecare, 6*, 63–72.

U.S. Department of Commerce (2002). *A nation online: How Americans are expanding their use of the Internet.* Washington, DC: U.S. Government Printing Office.

van Berlo, A. (1999). *Design guidelines on smart homes.* Available at: www.stakes.fi/cost219/smarthousing.htm

van Berlo, A. (2002). Smart home technology: Have older people paved the way? *Gerontechnology, 2*, 77–87.

Weiser, M. (1991). The computer for the 21st century. *Scientific American, 265*(3), 94–102.

2

Perceptual Aspects
of Gerotechnology

Charles T. Scialfa,
Geoffrey Ho, and
Jason Laberge

PERCEPTUAL ASPECTS OF GEROTECHNOLOGY

A variety of cognitive, affective, social, and cultural factors can render technologies more or less useful for older adults. Other contributors to this volume discuss many of these factors. This chapter focuses on aspects of sensory and perceptual aging that influence usability of current and emerging technologies. Emphasis is placed on vision, audition, and touch because technology is being used most regularly by the layperson in these modalities. Within this focus, coverage is directed toward areas of sensation and perception with the most obvious and direct use of technology. More extensive coverage of sensory and perceptual aging can be found in several recent reviews (e.g., Kline & Scialfa, 1997; Schneider & Pichora-Fuller, 2000). The chapter concludes with a consideration of two domains in which sensory and perceptual aging can influence the use of technology, in-vehicle telematics, and hand-held devices.

VISUAL PERCEPTION

Difficulties processing visual information are part of the aging process. Older adults report difficulties in spatial vision (acuity and contrast sensitivity), slowing of visual processing, seeing in poor light, seeing at near distances, and visual search (Kosnik, Winslow, Kline, Rasinski, & Sekuler, 1988; Rumsey, 1993). These difficulties are related to self-reported problems with driving (Kline, et al., 1992) and objective measures of functional vitality such as cessation of driving, distance judgments, and mobility (Kosnik, Sekuler, & Kline, 1990; Rubin, Roche, Prasada-Rao, & Fried, 1994). To explain the mechanisms that underlie these problems, we will briefly discuss the experimental data on visual function and age.

Age-related changes in pupil size reduce the amount of light reaching the retina, particularly at low light levels (Winn, Whitaker, Elliot, & Phillips, 1994). The older lens is more opaque and somewhat yellowed, reducing light further, particularly for short-wavelength colors like blue (Kashima, Trus, Unser, Edwards, & Datiles, 1993). The lens also loses its ability to change shape (i.e., accommodate) so as to bring objects to focus. This presbyopia increases blur for nearby objects and requires many older people to use multifocal lenses to see well under changing viewing distances. Light scatter within the older eye, attributable to changes in several optical structures, adds to image blur and decreases image contrast (van den Berg, 1995).

These structural changes influence perception most notably in spatial vision, as measured with acuity or contrast sensitivity. Acuity refers to the ability to see fine detail; contrast sensitivity is the ability to see small differences between the lightest and darkest parts of an image and is important when, for example, one must detect a truck on a foggy road.

Declines in acuity and contrast sensitivity are common in older adults (Gittings & Fozard, 1986; Scialfa, Adams, & Giovanetto, 1991). Age deficits in spatial vision are more pronounced as detail increases, under dynamic viewing conditions (Long & Crambert; 1990; Scialfa, Garvey, Tyrrell, & Leibowitz, 1992), after exposure to glare (Schieber & Kline, 1994), and when objects are closely spaced. Age deficits can be reduced, but not eliminated, with increased light and proper optical correction. It is also important to note that the optical corrections used by older adults reduce image blur only when the wearer is at the appropriate distance. Thus, bifocal lenses may be designed to provide the wearer with good acuity at 45 cm and at optical infinity (6 m), but objects viewed at other distances will be imaged with varying amounts of blur.

The implications are straightforward: If visual information is crowded by other stimuli, moving too quickly, presented at low contrast, in small print, or at the wrong viewing distance, older adults will have more difficulty using that information. They will have to make compensatory head and body movements to reduce image blur or will rely on a degraded image. The consequences are reduced accuracy, increased latency, and exacerbated visual fatigue.

An abundance of visual information outside of central vision can guide attention and eye movements, facilitate postural stability, and influence the perception of object and self-motion. Increasingly, computer-based tasks such as use of the Web, virtual reality, and vehicular telematics make use of spatially extended displays. Thus, age differences in peripheral vision will influence the ease with which these technologies are used.

Age deficits in acuity are greater for peripheral vision (Collins, Brown, & Bowman, 1989), and visual fields are reduced from approximately 180 degrees to 140 degrees by age 70 (Johnson, 1986). Further, several studies have demonstrated age-related reduction in the useful field of view (UFOV), the task-dependent spatial extent over which information can be extracted (Ball, Beard, Roenker, Miler, & Griggs, 1988; Scialfa, Kline, & Lyman, 1987). These restrictions can predict age-related risk of accident involvement (Owsley, Ball, Sloane, Roenker, & Bruni, 1991) and asymptotic age differences in simple visual search (Anandam & Scialfa, 1999).

When objects fall outside the UFOV, eye movements are required to process a scene. Thus, it is not surprising that older adults make more eye movements when searching through both simple and complex displays (Ho & Scialfa, 2002; Ho, Scialfa, Caird, & Graw, 2001; McPhee, Scialfa, Dennis, Ho, & Caird, in press; Scialfa, Thomas, & Joffe, 1994). Enhancement of figure-ground segregation, reduction in clutter, and consistency in target characteristics and location in particular can all reduce the need for eye movements and aid older users.

Color is critical to our use of visual space. Color differences across a scene facilitate the separation of figure and ground. Color differences are often quite salient and are rapidly used to discriminate and identify objects. Color imparts aesthetic value as well. The use of color in computer-based technology was uncommon a generation ago. Not so today.

For both neural and optical reasons that are only partially understood, older adults have some reliable difficulties processing color information. Shorter wavelengths, corresponding to the blue range of the visible spectrum, are more difficult to discriminate, especially in poor illumination (Cooper, Ward, Gowland, & McIntosh, 1991). If subtle color differences are used indiscriminately in technological applications, older adults will find them less accessible.

Most visual tasks require that attention be deployed to them in order to optimize performance. Attentional allocation may be involuntary, as with a sudden-onset warning, but often requires effortful, time-consuming, and sustained preparedness to respond to task-relevant information when more than one task is being performed. If older adults lack attentional resources or inefficiently distribute them, then performance will suffer. Does the literature on aging and attention suggest that this is likely? As in many cases, the answer to this question is not a simple one and depends on both attentional and nonattentional demands of the task (Madden & Whiting, 2003; McDowd & Shaw, 2000).

Consider some relatively automatic components of attention. The benefits associated with valid cueing of target location are equivalent or even greater for the elderly (Hartley, Kieley, & Slabach, 1990; Madden, 1992). However, consistent with a deficit in inhibitory control, attentional capture following the presentation of abrupt peripheral onsets or singletons appears to be greater among the elderly (Lincourt, Folk, & Hoyer, 1997; Pratt & Bellomo, 1999). Location-based inhibition of return, the slowing of response when targets appear at a previously attended position is slower to develop in the elderly (Castel, Chasteen, Scialfa, & Pratt, 2003) but is of equivalent magnitude (Hartley & Kieley, 1995). Priming of pop-out (Maljkovic & Nakayama, 2000) an implicit, facilitative effect of repeating a target's features (e.g., location or color), appears to be age-resistant (McCarley, Kramer, Colcombe, & Scialfa, 2003).

Other data suggest that some voluntary components of attentional allocation do not decline with age. Older adults' ability to sustain attention in vigilance tasks is not compromised when signal strength is sufficient (Giambra & Quilter, 1988) and there are no age differences in the ability to selectively attend to target features in order to automatize simple visual search tasks (Ho & Scialfa, 2002; Scialfa, Jenkins, Hamaluk, & Skaloud, 2000). Conversely, age deficits in vigilance emerge when signals are degraded (Parasuraman, Nestor, & Greenwood, 1989) and older adults have more difficulty in visual search when clutter, target-distractor complexity or similarity is increased (Plude & Doussard-Roosevelt, 1989, Scialfa, Esau, & Joffe, 1998). To a first approximation, it seems that age differences in lab-based tasks requiring voluntary attentional allocation increase with task complexity.

Even this seemingly safe conclusion may be an oversimplification. Most lab tasks have minimal allowances for the use of top-down processes that depend on context and experience. In addition, older adults may optimize performance on critical tasks by the strategic allocation of diminishing resources. These possibilities are illustrated in studies of visual search for traffic signs carried out in our lab. McPhee, Scialfia, Dennis, Ho, and Caird (in press) gave younger and older observers the task of searching for traffic signs. They carried out these searches as a single task and when engaged in a secondary verbal task. There were no age differences in search performance, but older adults remembered very little of the verbal material under the dual-task conditions. Karen Li and her colleagues have reported that for very different tasks, older adults can prioritize multiple tasks and shed those deemed less important (Li, Lindenberger, Freund, & Baltes, 2001). Thus, if technologies are designed to allow this sort of strategic task-switching, age differences in primary task performance may be minimized.

Ours is a dynamic world, in which objects move with varying speeds, in all directions, amidst other objects. The accurate perception of motion influences diverse processes including the execution of eye movements, figure-ground segregation, the deployment of attention, and the anticipation of actions such as reaching, postural stability, and locomotion. Any technology for the elderly that makes use of motion or is used in dynamic environments should consider age-related changes in motion perception.

A relatively small literature on the topic leads to the view that thresholds for simple motion stimuli are elevated in older people (Atchley & Andersen, 1998; Gilmore, Wenk, Naylor, & Stuve, 1992). At a behavioral level, there are age deficits in using optical flow to detect three-dimensional surfaces (Andersen & Atchley, 1995) and in reaction time to motion onset (Porciatti, Fiorentini, Morrone, & Burr, 1999). Scialfa, Guzy, Leibowitz, Garvey, and Tyrrell (1991) observed small but consistent age differences in the ability to estimate vehicle velocity, and Andersen, Cisneros, Saidpour, and Atchley (2000) reported that older observers were less able to avoid simulated collisions using information about their rate of deceleration. In visual search, Folk & Lincourt (1996) found that the elderly made less effective use of coherent motion to optimize search, but Kramer, Martin-Emerson, Larish, and Andersen (1996) detected no age differences in the ability to use movement to filter relevant from irrelevant objects.

Obviously, additional research is needed in this area. Despite the theoretical importance of age differences in motion perception under tightly controlled experimental conditions, they may not generalize to everyday tasks (Andersen & Atchley, 1995). In addition, because motion perception can be based on multiple visual, proprioceptive, and vestibular inputs, it is unlikely that motion differences in one task will generalize to different tasks. Finally, we know very little about age differences in motion perception in constructed environments such as simulators and virtual spaces, even though the immediate future will involve their greater use.

AUDITORY PERCEPTION

Hearing loss is a problem frequently observed and reported in older people (Haber, 1994). When elders are asked about their everyday problems involving hearing, those most commonly reported involve slowing of auditory processing, hearing in noisy environments, understanding both normal and distorted speech, and hearing sounds of higher frequency (Slawinski, Hartel, & Kline, 1993). Technology may exacerbate these problems because sound is being used as a means of communication under temporally demanding and noisy conditions where signal distortions are likely. Consider, for example, using text-to-speech applications to allow for receipt of e-mail while driving. Speech compression algorithms will increase temporal processing demands and shift the signal to higher frequencies. In addition, the speech signal will need to be extracted from road and engine noise, passenger conversations, radio broadcasts, etc. How will older listeners cope with these compromised signals? Both peripheral and more central changes in auditory processing suggest that they will face numerous challenges.

Structural changes within the peripheral auditory system are well known. The auditory canal becomes more susceptible to collapse when earphones are worn, reducing transmission of high-frequency sound (Schow & Goldblum, 1980). The eardrum loses its elasticity, resulting in a reduction in signal strength and the small bones of the middle ear also become calcified, diminishing signal amplitude further (Etholm & Belal, 1974). Changes to the inner ear and auditory nerve also reduce hearing (Matschke, 1990; Ryals & Westbrook, 1988).

The ability to hear simple tones shows reliable age declines (Gates, Cooper, Kannel, & Miller, 1990) that are most pronounced at higher frequencies. This phenomenon, known as presbycusis, is greater for men than women (Pedersen, Rosenhall, & Moller, 1989). However, there is some evidence that gender differences in hearing loss may reverse at low frequencies (Jerger, Chmiel, Stach, & Spretnjak, 1993) and this can have implications for the use of low frequencies as warning signals.

While signal strength can be increased using amplification at the sound source or hearing aids, many such devices amplify all signals including noise, an effect that prompts older listeners to discontinue their use (Pichora-Fuller, 1997). Programmable hearing aids can be used to selectively amplify frequencies in the speech range and even to differentially enhance signals coming from particular locations relative to the listener. Unfortunately, older people often have a poor understanding of how these devices operate and so may not be able to use them effectively. One area in which technology can be used to reduce this problem is by providing interactive training in the intelligent use of these devices.

The ability to discriminate among frequencies is important to speech perception and is compromised in older adults (Abel, Krever, & Alberti, 1990); while greater at high frequencies problems also occur at low frequencies (Moore & Peters, 1992). Although the high-frequency losses may be attributable, in part, to changes in absolute thresholds, the low frequency declines are likely central in origin, perhaps due to loss of temporal synchrony in old age.

Temporal sensitivity is also critical to the perception of complex auditory signals such as speech and music. Several studies have found that temporal resolution is reduced in old age (e.g., Schneider, Speranza, & Pichora-Fuller, 1998). Losses in temporal sensitivity persist when puretone hearing loss is controlled, suggesting a more central cause. Consequently, older adults are less able to use interaural differences to isolate a signal from noise (Grose, Poth, & Peters, 1994; Pichora-Fuller & Schneider, 1991), with an impact on localization, speech recognition in noise, and auditory scene analysis.

A great deal of auditory perception requires that attention be allocated efficiently and appropriately to the task. In speech recognition, for example, the ability to isolate relevant from irrelevant auditory streams requires heightened activation of some input channels and inhibition of others. In other cases, processing of auditory signals must occur in environments where attention is divided among multiple signals, often across multiple sensory modalities. Self-report data (Tun & Wingfield, 1995) indicate that older adults experience divided attention involving auditory signals, such as talking while playing cards. Does the experimental literature substantiate these subjective data?

Attentionally mediated filtering of irrelevant information appears to be identical for younger and older adults (Ison, Virag, Allen, & Hammond, 2002). In addition, when adjustments are made for hearing losses, older adults do not have greater difficulty inhibiting the processing of auditory distractors (Hugdahl, Carlsson, & Eichele, 2001) although they may show deficits when more effortful processing is demanded (Amenedo & Diaz, 1998). When Hawkins, Kramer, and Capaldi (1992) asked a life-span adult sample to carry out a choice reaction time (RT) task that alternated between visual and auditory inputs, they found task-switching produced costs for all people, but more so for the older adults. Speech processing under dual-task conditions is also disproportionately reduced in the elderly (Tun, Wingfield, & Stine, 1991).

Thus far we have discussed several changes in the auditory system and in hearing that would be expected to influence speech perception, but we have not dealt with age differences in speech recognition per se. Numerous studies indicate that older adults have difficulties with speech recognition, which are magnified when the speech is presented in noisy or reverberant environments (Abel, Krever, & Alberti, 1990; van Rooj & Plomp, 1992). Clearly, it is unlikely that amplification alone will compensate for all of the difficulties encountered by older adults in understanding speech.

There are two ways that we know speech perception can be enhanced in the elderly. The first involves the appropriate use of context. Relative to the young, older adults make as much or more use of semantic context to facilitate speech recognition (Craig, Kim, Rhyner, & Chirillo, 1993), perhaps reflecting their continuing use of and expertise with language (Tun & Wingfield, 1995). Developers might be tempted to reduce context by using abbreviated messages when presenting speech signals in their applications. This is likely to work to the detriment of older listeners.

The second method is through appropriate modification of the complexity, enunciation, and timing of the speech signal. Clear Speech, a trainable technique for enhancing speech recognition in the hearing-impaired, can work well for older listeners, too, but it is important to ensure that Clear Speech does not devolve to "elderspeak" (Kemper & Lacal, 2003), a semantically simplified and affectively patronizing communicative style that is offensive to many older listeners and detracts from speech comprehension.

TOUCH AND MOVEMENT

Older adults manifest a loss of sensation in various parts of the body including the feet, lips, fingers, and the fleshy area below the thumb. These include declines in sensitivity to pressure (Kenshalo, 1986), vibration (Gescheider, Beiles, Checkosky, Bolanowski, & Verrillo, 1994), spatial acuity (Stevens & Cruz, 1996), and the perception of roughness, length, and orientation (Stevens & Patterson, 1995). Sensory decline is found in healthy older adults, but is more pronounced in a number of age-related diseases including Parkinson's disease (Sathian, Zangaladze, Green, Vitek, & DeLong, 1997).

In addition to these sensory deficits, changes in the joints and bones of the hand reduce grip strength and range of motion (Carmeli, Patish, & Coleman, 2003). Many older adults, especially those with arthritic conditions, have difficulty with technology-mediated motor tasks like keyboard entry (Chaparro, Rogers, Fernandez, Bohan, Choi, et al., 2000). In addition, age-related changes in muscle composition and activation are important determinants of difficulties with motor control. All types of muscle fibers decrease with age, but the reductions are most pronounced for fast-twitch fibers (Fiatarone Singh, et al., 1999). There is also a loss and reorganization of motor units that reduces the smoothness and coordination of movements (Roos, Rice, & Vandervoort, 1997).

As might be expected then, movement time, defined as the interval between the initiation and ending of movement, increase for a variety of point-to-point and continuous movements, particularly large movements (Ketcham, Seidler, Van Gemmert, & Stelmach, 2002). Forces used to move are more "jumpy" (Brown, 1996), peak velocity is lower (Pratt, Chasteen & Abrams, 1994), and the deceleration phase, where corrective action can be taken, is disproportionately lengthened (Brown, 1996). Older adults also make more secondary, corrective movements to a target. As might be expected, coordinating multiple movements (e.g., required for reaching to grasp or typing show marked declines (Ketcham, Seidler, Van Gemmert, & Stelmach, 2002).

COMMON ISSUES FOR HAND-HELD
DEVICES AND IN-VEHICLE TELEMATICS

Computers are starting to look much less like the traditional desktop workstation. Tasks that once were available only on desktop PCs are being performed on hand-held devices or on systems that are embedded within our homes and cars. Hand-held devices, several of which are shown in Figure 2.1, generally refer to self-contained systems that can be used and manipulated while being held. They include commonly use products like cellular telephones and personal digital assistants (PDAs), but also in-home medical devices such as monitors for glucose levels and location monitors that allow caregivers to supervise children or seniors from a distance.

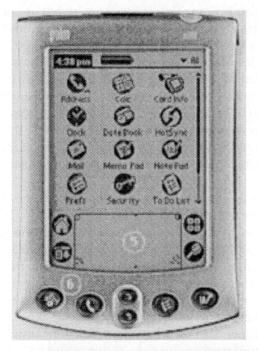
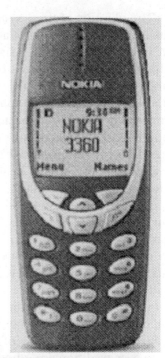
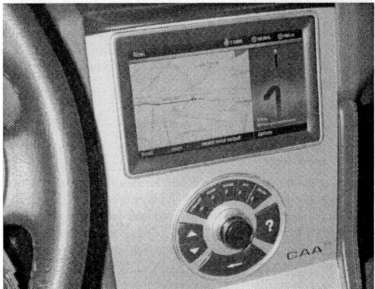

FIGURE 2.1 Examples of Currently Available Hand-held (Upper Panels) and Telematics (Lower Panel) Devices.

The ubiquity of these systems is not trivial. It is estimated that about 46–50% of households in Canada and the U.S. have a cellular phone and in some European and Asian nations the numbers approach 80–90% (Ipsos-Reid, 2001). PDAs are less common. Currently only 8% of households in the United States own one, but the potential of these devices may equal that of laptop computing (Ipsos-Reid, 2001). Portable health care devices are also expected to become more popular. With an aging population, the increasing pressure to reduce health care costs, and the trend for the public to take a more active role in their own health care, technology for home health care has become a growth industry (Rousseau & Nunes, 2002).

Another emerging trend is the development of in-vehicle telematics for automobiles, also shown in Figure 2.1. Telematics refers to a wide variety of safety, entertainment, diagnostic, office, and traffic information technologies. Presently, advanced telematics systems only exist in luxury automobiles, and even then there is limited functionality, but this will change. These devices have promising potential to enable older adults to continue productive and independent lifestyles. However, older adults still lack the confidence to use such systems, have less knowledge and understanding of them, and feel that they offer little advantage over traditional methods of performing tasks (Kline, Caird, Ho, & Dewar, 2002). To encourage an older population to use them, they must be adequately designed to meet the sensory and perceptual changes of senescence. In the following section, we will examine how many of these devices perform in this regard and how they can be designed to allow for better usability.

VISUAL PERCEPTION

Visual Acuity

Both hand-held devices and in-vehicle telematics rely primarily on a traditional graphical user interface (GUI) to present information. However, because these systems are portable and used in diverse environments, they present new problems in design for older adults. Most notable is the reduced screen size and resolution of these displays. A typical cell phone, for example, has a resolution of 96 x 65 pixels (3G Lab, 2002) and a typical PDA displays information at 240 x 320 pixels (Kärkkäinen & Laarni, 2002). Because of the limitations on resolution and screen size, designers often compact great amounts of information by miniaturizing and crowding text and graphics, thus requiring users to have relatively good acuity in order to use the device. This problem is magnified because inexpensive PDAs and cell phones still have low contrast monochrome screens that may reduce legibility. Kärkkäinen and Laarni (2002) found that the poorer resolution of PDAs resulted in worse performance on an information retrieval task for younger adults; undoubtedly, the retrieval problems would be even greater for a presbyopic older adult who may not have 20/20 near vision.

Optical blur is another problem for in-vehicle telematic displays. Although these displays are generally larger and have higher resolution, they are presented at a fixed distance, usually somewhere between 65—85 cm. Because many older adults wear bifocals, objects are only in focus at optical infinity, approximately 45 cm. Thus, optical blur may be considerable and high frequency information will be lost.

Kline and colleagues (2002) assessed some currently available in-vehicle navigational displays and found they had several acuity-related problems. Of the vehicles examined, they found that only one vehicle manufacturer used fonts that were adequate for the viewing distance of 65 cm, and none of the assessed navigational displays used fonts that were adequate for 85 cm. Additionally, Kline and colleagues (2002) showed how, with increasing age, the ability to accommodate to objects at 65–85 cm becomes more difficult when viewed through a far-distance optical correction and a near-distance optical correction. The average 52-year-old would be unable to properly focus on an object at the critical viewing distances with either a far or near correction.

Progressive lenses can compensate for the inability to accommodate to intermediate distances. However, many older adults do not use these lenses and even when they do, there are problems associated with them. From a design perspective, at least two options are available. First, placing screens closer, such as in the dash window or slightly above the steering wheel, would bring the viewing distance closer to 40 cm. Or, screens could be placed on an adjustable arm to allow users to manipulate viewing distance. Second, increasing font size and graphic size does help comprehension and reading speed. Kärkkäinen and Laarni (2002) recommend that 14 pt. fonts should be used for PDAs even for younger adult users. Therefore, 16 pt. fonts may be more appropriate for older adults. Omori, Watanabe, Takai, Takada, and Miyao (2002) found that by increasing the font size of mobile phones, both older and younger adults increased their reading speed and made significantly fewer errors. Similarly, guidelines for navigational displays (e.g., Cambell, Carney, &

Kantowitz, 1998) suggest that fonts should be at least between .27–.45° of visual angle, which corresponds to approximately 20–26 pt. Arial type at 85cm. However, because screen "real estate" is limited, increasing the size of text and objects comes at a cost. If the size of text and objects is increased, users will either be forced to scroll or go through multiple menus to find needed information, or developers will need to consider eliminating unnecessary options and functions.

Environmental Illumination

Unlike desktop computers that are used indoors, portable devices and in-vehicle telematics are often viewed in sunlight, which can reduce legibility, or in places where there is very little light, such as while sitting in the back seat of a car at night. In this case, the lack of light makes it difficult to use the device. The dynamic nature of the lighting situation (e.g., driving in and out of sun and shade) can make matters worse. Because older adults take longer for light and dark adaptation, are more susceptible to the effects of glare, and because their vision suffers more in low luminance conditions, steps to counter the effects of external light sources (or lack thereof) are important.

In bright sunlight hand-held devices have an advantage over fixed in-vehicle telematics displays near the windshield because the glare can often be reduced by shielding, or by holding the device at a different angle. However, fixed telematic screens can be designed using the same defenses against glare such as embedding the screen in an outer hood (U.S. Department of Defense, 1989), or adding a tilt feature on the screen. Lastly, designers can add antiglare filters. Somewhat ironically, the brightness of in-vehicle telematics displays themselves can be a source of distraction and can interfere with on-road visibility. Better-designed displays offer automatic dimming functions that adjust the screen luminance to cabin light levels. Another solution to reduce the effects of bright displays at night is to use reverse polarity displays.

In low light conditions, the simplest method to increase legibility is to provide easy access controls that allow the user to adjust the screen's luminance and contrast. Although most hand-held devices offer this option, these controls are often buried deep in menus in the interface itself, making them difficult to access. Some hand-held devices also take advantage of reversing polarity to aid low luminance conditions; however, the legibility is reduced when using reverse polarity on devices that rely on a monochrome screen (Muter, 1996). A final way that hand-held devices and telematic displays overcome low luminance conditions is by providing backlighting for their controls. Most cellular phones are armed with this capability, but many of the hard buttons on PDAs do not come with this feature.

Color

The color capabilities of hand-held devices are improving. For example, advanced PDAs are capable of displaying up to 65,000 colors. While color perception for older adults does not appear to be seriously impaired, there are subtle differences that may affect an older adult's ability to process visual information (Kline & Scialfa, 1997). In particular, the ability to distinguish between short-wavelength colors such as violet, blue, and green is reduced in the elderly. Thus, small icons and graphics that contain low color contrast steps between short-wavelength colors will not likely be very visible to the older eye. In addition, color coding may be less effective if many of the color codes are short-wavelength colors. Therefore, if low contrast steps are to be used or color coding is used, longer-wavelength colors (i.e., yellow, red, and orange) are recommended.

Display Layout

As products (and displays) continue to shrink, presenting large amounts of information simultaneously will increase visual clutter. Several interface design guidelines suggest that if information is to be presented on a small display, the amount of information presented should be reduced (Jones, Marsden, Mohd-Nasir, Boone, & Buchanan, 1999). Methods that have been developed to reduce search demands on the Web should also apply to hand-held devices and in-vehicle telematics. For instance, frequently used items should be placed near the top of a menu. In addition, consistent layouts will provide the user with improved ability to find what they are looking for. Critical items and titles will benefit from high color contrast and increased font size relative to the noncritical items in the display.

AUDITORY PERCEPTION

Although a great deal of information is presented visually, for some devices like cellular phones and music players the transmission of sound is the primary method of communication. PDAs also use auditory alerts to notify users of an upcoming event and some health monitors send an auditory alarm when a safety parameter has been exceeded. Sounds are also used in more subtle ways to provide feedback that an action has occurred. In more advanced systems, voice recognition software interprets human voice commands and digitized speech is used to respond. Given that many older adults have hearing impairments, devices that utilize auditory output need to consider their limitations. Unfortunately, there is a paucity of research examining auditory factors and usability of computerized devices. Thus, there are many issues that need to be addressed.

Many of us have now used a cellular phone and are familiar with its advantages. However, we are also familiar with the common breakdown in the quality of the voice transmission. The reasons for this depend on a variety of factors. The common analog cellular phone is actually a radio, thus all the situations that interfere with radio signals, such as driving through a tunnel, can affect the quality of the transmission. Analog phones are comparable to wired telephones in voice quality because they use the same range of frequencies to transmit a signal (Farley & Van der Hoek, 2002). Wired telephones eliminate sounds below 400 Hz and sounds above 3400 Hz, which corresponds quite closely to the range of human speech (550–5000Hz) (Kline & Scialfa, 1997). The sound quality of digital phones can be much better, because digital technology reproduces the original sound much better. However, digital signals are also compressed, meaning that they too may have certain frequencies eliminated to save on bandwidth. Moreover, although digital technology uses a smaller bandwidth for transmission, telephone companies use this to their advantage and try to put as many users in a channel as possible. As more users occupy the channel bandwidth, the quality of the transmission deteriorates (Farley & Van der Hoek, 2002). A reduction in sound quality of cellular phones is also the result of environmental noise. Unlike home phones that are often used in relative quiet, cellular phones are often used in very noisy environments.

These problems are annoying even to the average younger user, thus it is likely that any reduction of sound quality will affect an older person's perceived usability of a device. The detection of high frequency sounds (such as are needed to discriminate 's' and 'f') will likely be impaired (Kline & Scialfa, 1997), as would the detection of high-frequency tones and beeps that are presented too quietly. Simple methods to overcome these problems include easy access to volume controls and using lower-frequency sounds for tones, beeps, and rings.

3G cellular technologies, which allow for a greater bandwidth and fast, wireless transmission of data, promise to overcome some of the voice quality problems experienced with current cellular phones. Users will also be able to incorporate video with voice transmissions on a cellular device. This would allow users to use visual cues such as gesture and expressions to aid speech perception, although the quality of the video would have to be quite good for it to be effective (Charness, 2001).

Ambient noise is also a concern when it is presented inside a vehicle, since many in-vehicle telematics incorporate cellular phone calls as a hands-free option. With advances in wireless and voice technology, hands-free voice interactions will likely be common in the future. However, cabin and traffic noise can degrade the auditory message (Dahl & Claesson, 1996). The signal of both the driver's voice and any computer-generated speech must be strong enough to be heard through this. Computer generated speech may be more problematic for older drivers, not only because of noise, but also because it lacks the prosody and inflections used in normal speech that aid speech comprehension (Kiss & Ennis, 2001).

TOUCH AND MOVEMENT

A final concern with hand-held devices is the difficulty older adults may have manipulating the stylus, buttons, and dials. Arthritis and tremors, more prevalent among the older populations, make it difficult to perform fine motor movements. Yet most hand-held devices, due to their smaller size, require fine, discrete movements to tap very small targets (e.g., the keys of a virtual keyboard), to press small buttons, or to write with a stylus. The knobs and buttons also give little tactile feedback to indicate that they have been scrolled or depressed. Many cell phones also have a vibratory alert to indicate a call is coming in. While it is unknown whether older adults have more trouble responding to this sort of alarm, it is known that older adults have a higher threshold for vibratory detection (Goble, Collins, & Cholewiak, 1996).

While in-vehicle telematics do not generally rely on tactile output, fine motor movements are still needed because some require manipulating the controls. Finally, reaching motions are a concern for in-vehicle telematics because many older adults find reaching to be painful, which limits their ability to execute quick manipulations with arm movements. Thus, keeping device controls closer to the older driver to avoid extensive reach is important. Moving large buttons closer or placing some controls on the steering wheel may alleviate reach problems.

FUTURE DIRECTIONS

Although technology can greatly aid older adults, it must first be designed to accommodate their needs. Yet, we still know very little about how to do this effectively. There is a great need for both basic and applied research to address the usability of devices for the aged. Many of the problems and design solutions addressed above are still speculative and are based on the psychophysics of the older adult's sensory and perceptual system. But, much of this basic psychological research is dated, has a bias towards visual processes, and focuses on addressing the limits of the sensory system. Although this research may have important psychological significance, it does not always address the concerns that are confronted by designers and engineers.

Even when guidelines are developed that are shown to improve design, they often are not followed. Guidelines are often vague because the correct design solution depends on the situation in which the device will be used. In order for this information to be useful, it must be presented in a fashion such that those designing the product are able to use it and understand it. One reason why this is so difficult to achieve is because there is dissociation between those of us who are in psychology and those who are in medicine, engineering, computer science, and other disciplines associated with technology design.

In this chapter, an attempt was made to look into the near future of computing and address how the limitations of the older sensory and perceptual system might affect the usability of emerging devices. At times, clear solutions can be provided, but at other times there is simply not enough research available to provide any obvious solutions. This may be the most important point to be made in this chapter. Much research is needed. This research needs to be focused on both basic sensory systems of the older adult (particularly in audition and haptics) and their effect on using technology. Because technology seems to move much faster than our ability to produce this information, it makes sense to look forward at emerging technologies in order to keep pace, and there is a greater need to incorporate an interdisciplinary approach so that those who are designing and building the technologies are able to use this information.

ACKNOWLEDGMENTS

Charles T. Scialfa, Geoffrey Ho, and Jason Laberge work in the Perception, Aging, and Cognitive Ergonomics Program, Department of

Psychology, University of Calgary. Their work was supported by a grant from the Natural Science and Engineering Research Council of Canada. Requests for reprints should be addressed to C. T. (Chip) Scialfa, Department of Psychology, University of Calgary, Calgary, AB T2N 1N4, CANADA. E-mail: scialfa@ucalgary.ca.

REFERENCES

3G Lab (2002, October). The total handset user experience: A technical white paper.

Abel, S., Krever, E., & Alberti, P. (1990). Auditory detection, discrimination, and speech processing in ageing, noise-sensitive and hearing-impaired listeners. *Scandinavian Audiology, 19,* 43–54.

Amenedo, E., & Diaz, F. (1998). Automatic and effortful processes in auditory memory reflected by event-related potentials: Age-related findings. *Electroencephalography and Clinical Neurophysiology: Evoked Potentials, 108,* 361–369.

Anandam, B., & Scialfa, C. (1999). Aging and the development of automaticity in feature search. *Aging, Neuropsychology, and Cognition, 6,* 117–140.

Andersen, G., & Atchley, P. (1995). Age-related differences in the detection of three-dimensional surfaces from optic flow. *Psychology and Aging, 10,* 650–658.

Andersen, G., Cisneros, J., Saidpour, A., & Atchley, P. (2000). Age-related differences in collision detection during deceleration. *Psychology and Aging, 15,* 241–252.

Atchley, P., & Andersen, G. (1998). The effect of age, retinal eccentricity, and speed on the detection of optic flow components. *Psychology and Aging, 13,* 297–308.

Ball, K., Beard, B., Roenker, D., Miler, R., & Griggs, D. (1988). Age and visual search: Expanding the useful field of view. *Journal of the Optical Society of America A, 35,* 2210–2219.

Brown, S. (1996). Control of simple arm movements in the elderly. In A. M. Fernandez & N. Teasdale (Eds.), *Changes in sensory motor behavior in aging.* Amsterdam: Elsevier Science.

Cambell, J. L., Carney, C., & Kantowitz, B. H. (1998). *Human factors design guidelines for advanced traveler information systems (ATIS) and commercial vehicle operations (CVO).* McLean, VA: Federal Highway Association.

Carmeli, E., Patish, H., & Coleman, R. (2003). The aging hand. *Journals of Gerontology Series A: Biological and Medical Sciences, 58A,* 146–152.

Castel, A., Chasteen, A., Scialfa, C., & Pratt, J. (2003). *Adult age differences in the time course of inhibition of return. Journals of Gerontology Series B: Psychological Sciences and Social Sciences, 58B,* 256–260.

Chaparro, A., Rogers, M., Fernandez, J., Bohan, M., Choi, S., & Stumpfhauser, L. (2000). Range of motion for the wrist: Implications for designing computer input devices for the elderly. *Disability Rehabilitation, 22,* 633–637.

Charness, N. (2001). Aging and communication: Human factors issues. In N. Charness, D. C. Park, & B. A. Sabel (Eds.), *Communication, technology, and aging: Opportunities and challenges for the future.* New York: Springer Publishing.

Collins, M. J., Brown, B., & Bowman, K. J. (1989). Peripheral visual acuity and age. *Ophthalmic and Physiological Optics, 9,* 314–316.

Cooper, B., Ward, M., Gowland, C., & McIntosh, J., (1991). The use of the Lanthony New Color Test in determining the effects of aging on color vision. *Journal of Gerontology: Psychological Sciences, 46,* 320–324.

Craig, C., Kim, B., Rhyner, P., & Chirillo, T. (1993). Effects of word predictability, child development, and aging on time-gated speech recognition performance. *Journal of Speech and Hearing Research, 36,* 832–841.

Dahl, M., & Claesson, I. (1996). A neural network trained microphone array system for noise reduction. *Proceedings of the IEEE Signal Processing Society Workshop on Neural Networks for Signal Processing,* Japan.

Etholm, B., & Belal, A. (1974). Senile changes in the middle ear joints. *Annals of Otology, Rhinology and Laryngology, 83,* 49–64.

Farley, T., & Van der Hoek, M. (2002). Cellular phone basics: AMPS and beyond. Retrieved March 25, 2003 from www.privateline.com/Cellbasics/ Cellbasics.html

Fiatarone Singh, M. A., Ding, W., Manfredi, T. J., Solares, G., O'Neill, E. F., Clements, K. M., et al. (1999). Insulin-like growth factor I in skeletal muscle after weight-lifting exercise in frail elders. *American Journal of Physiology: Endocrinology and Metabolism, 40,* E135—E143.

Folk, C., & Lincourt, A. (1996). The effects of age on guided conjunction search. *Experimental Aging Research, 22,* 99–118.

Gates, G., Cooper, J., Kannel, W., & Miller, N. (1990). Hearing in the elderly: The Framingham cohort, 1983–1985: Part I. Basic audiometric test results. *Ear and Hearing, 11,* 247–256.

Gescheider, G. A., Beiles, E. J., Checkosky, C. M., Bolanowski, S. J., & Verrillo, R. T. (1994). The effects of aging on information-processing channels in the sense of touch: II. Temporal summation in the P channel. *Somatosensory and Motor Research, 11,* 359–365.

Giambra, L., & Quilter, R. (1988). Sustained attention in adulthood: A unique, large-sample, longitudinal and multicohort analysis using the Mackworth Clock-Test. *Psychology & Aging, 3,* 75–83.

Gilmore, G., Wenk, H., Naylor, L., & Stuve, T. (1992). Motion perception and aging. *Psychology and Aging, 7,* 654–660.

Gittings, N., & Fozard, J. (1986). Age changes in visual acuity. *Experimental Gerontology, 21,* 423–434.

Goble, A. K., Collins, A. A., & Cholewiak, R. W. (1996). Vibrotactile threshold in young and old observers: The effects of spatial summation and the presence of a rigid surround. *Journal of the Acoustical Society of America, 99,* 2256–2269.

Grose, J., Poth, E., & Peters, R. (1994). Masking level differences for tones and speech in elderly listeners with relatively normal audiograms. *Speech & Hearing Research, 37,* 422–428.

Haber, D. (1994). *Health promotion and aging.* New York: Springer Publishing.

Hartley, A. A., & Kieley, J. M. (1995). Adult age difference in the inhibition of return of visual attention. *Psychology and Aging, 10,* 670–683.

Hartley, A. A., Kieley, J. M., & Slabach, E. H. (1990). Age differences and similarities in the effects of cues and prompts. *Journal of Experimental Psychology: Human Perception and Performance, 16,* 523–537.

Hawkins, H., Kramer, A., & Capaldi, D. (1992). Aging, exercise, and attention. *Psychology and Aging, 7,* 643–653.

Ho, G., & Scialfa, C. T. (2002). Age, skill transfer and conjunction search. *Journal of Gerontology: Psychological Sciences, 57B,* 277–287.

Ho, G., Scialfa, C., Caird, J., & Graw, T. (2001). Conspicuity of traffic signs: The effect of clutter, luminance and aging. *Human Factors, 43,* 194–207.

Hugdahl, K., Carlsson, G., & Eichele, T. (2001). Age effects in dichotic listening to consonant-vowel syllables: Interactions with attention. *Developmental Neuropsychology, 20,* 445–457

Ison, J., Virag, T., Allen, P., & Hammond, G. (2002). The attention filter for tones in noise has the same shape and effective bandwidth in the elderly as it has in young listeners. *Journal of the Acoustical Society of America, 112,* 238–245.

Ipsos-Reid (2001). On the run with technology. *World Monitor, 2,* 26–34.

Jerger, J., Chmiel, R., Stach, B., & Spretnjak, M. (1993). Gender affects audiometric shape in presbycusis. *Journal of the American Academy of Audiology, 4,* 42–49.

Johnson, C. (1986, February). *Peripheral visual fields and driving in an aging population.* Paper presented at the Invitational Conference on Work, Aging, and Vision, National Research Council, Washington, D.C.

Jones, M., Marsden, G., Mohd-Nasir, N., Boone, K., & Buchanan, G. (1999, May). Improving web interaction on small displays. Proceedings of the Eighth International Conference on the World Wide Web, Toronto, Canada, 1129–1137.

Kärkkäinen, L., & Laarni, J. (2002, October). Designing for small display screens. *Proceedings of the Second Nordic Conference on Human-Computer Interaction,* Aarhus, Denmark, 227–230.

Kashima, K., Trus, B., Unser, M., Edwards, P., & Datiles, M. (1993). Aging studies on normal lens using the Scheimpflug slit-lamp camera. *Investigative Ophthalmology and Visual Science, 334,* 293–26.

Kemper, S., & Lacal, J. (2003). Addressing the communication needs of an aging society. *Steering Committee: Workshop on Technology for Adaptive Aging.* National Research Council, January 23–25, Washington, D.C.

Kenshalo, D. (1986). Somesthetic sensitivity in young and elderly humans. *Journal of Gerontology, 41,* 732–742.

Ketcham, C., Seidler, R., Van Gemmert, A., & Stelmach, G. (2002). Age related kinematic differences as influenced by task difficulty, target-size, and movement amplitude. *Journal of Gerontology: Psychological Sciences, 57B,* 54–64.

Kiss, I., & Ennis, T. (2001). Age-related decline in perception of prosodic affect. *Applied Neuropsychology, 8,* 251–254.

Kline, D., Caird, J. K., Ho, G., & Dewar, R. E. (2002). *Analytic study to assess the visual deficits of aging drivers and the legibility of on-board intelligent transport systems (ITS) displays.* (T8080—011146/001/SS). Ottawa, ON: Transport Canada.

Kline, D., Kline T., Fozard, J., Kosnik, W., Schieber, F., & Sekuler, R. (1992). Vision, aging and driving: The problems of older drivers. *Journal of Gerontology: Psychological Sciences, 47,* 27–43.

Kline, D. W., & Scialfa, C. T. (1997). Sensory and perceptual functioning: Basic research and human factors applications. In A. D. Fisk & W. A. Rogers (Eds.), *Handbook of human factors and the older adult.* San Diego: Academic.

Kosnik, W., Winslow, L., Kline, D., Rasinski, K., et al. (1988). Visual changes in daily life throughout adulthood. *Journal of Gerontology, 43,* P63-P70.

Kosnik, W., Sekuler, R., & Kline, D. (1990). Self-reported visual problems of older drivers. *Human Factors, 32,* 597–608

Kramer, A., Martin-Emerson, R., Larish, J., & Andersen, G. (1996). Aging and filtering by movement in visual search. *Journals of Gerontology Series B - Psychological Sciences and Social Sciences, 51,* P201—P216.

Li, K. Z. H., Lindenberger, U., Freund, A. M., & Baltes, P. B. (2001). Walking while memorizing: Age-related differences in compensatory behavior. *Psychological Science, 12,* 230–237.

Lincourt, A. E., Folk, C. L., & Hoyer, W. J. (1997). Effects of aging on voluntary and involuntary shifts of attention. *Aging, Neuropsychology and Cognition, 4,* 290–303.

Long, G., & Crambert, R. (1990). The nature and basis of age-related changes in dynamic visual acuity. *Psychology and Aging, 5,* 138–143.

Madden, D. (1992). Selective attention and visual search: Revision of an allocation model and application to age differences. *Journal of Experimental Psychology: Human Perception and Performance, 18,* 821–836.

Madden, D., & Whiting, W. (2003). Age-related changes in visual attention. In P. Costa & I. Siegler (Eds.), *Recent advances in psychology and aging.* Amsterdam: Elsevier.

Maljkovic, V., & Nakayama, K. (2000). Priming of popout: III. A short-term implicit memory system beneficial for rapid target selection. *Visual Cognition, 7,* 571–595.

Matschke, R. (1990). Frequency selectivity and psychoacoustic tuning curves in old age. *Acta Oto-Laryngologica, 476* (Supplement), 114–119.

McCarley, J., Kramer, A., Colcombe, A., & Scialfa, C. (2003). Priming of pop-out in visual search: A Comparison of young and old adults. Unpublished manuscript.

McDowd, J., & Shaw, R. (2000). Attention and aging: A functional perspective. In F. I. M. Craik & T. A. Salthouse (Eds.), *The handbook of aging and cognition* (2nd ed.). New York: Lawrence Erlbaum.

McPhee, L., Scialfa, C., Dennis, W., Ho, G., & Caird, J. (in press). Age differences in visual search for traffic signs under divided attention conditions. *Human Factors*.

Moore, B., & Peters, R. (1992). Pitch discrimination and phase sensitivity in young and elderly subjects and its relationship to frequency selectivity. *Journal of the Acoustical Society of America, 91*, 2881–2893.

Muter, P. (1996). Interface design and optimization of reading of continuous text. In H. van Oostendorp & S. de Mul (Eds.), *Cognitive aspects of electronic text processing*. Norwood, NJ: Ablex Publishing Corp.

Omori, M., Watanabe, T., Takai, J., Takada, H., & Miyao, M. (2002). Visibility and characteristics of the mobile phone for elderly people. *Behaviour and Information Technology, 21*, 313–316.

Owsley, C., Ball, K., Sloane, M., Roenker, D., & Bruni, J. (1991). Visual/cognitive correlates of vehicle accidents in older drivers. *Psychology and Aging, 6*, 403–415.

Parasuraman, R., Nestor, P., & Greenwood, P. (1989). Sustained-attention capacity in young and older adults. *Psychology and Aging, 4*, 339–345.

Pedersen, K., Rosenhall, U., & Moller, M. (1989). Changes in pure-tone thresholds in individuals aged 70–81: Results from a longitudinal study. *Audiology, 28*, 194–204.

Pichora-Fuller, M. (1997). Language comprehension in older listeners. *Journal of Speech Language Pathology and Audiology, 21*, 125–142.

Pichora-Fuller, M., & Schneider, B. (1991). Masking-level differences in the elderly: A comparison of antiphasic and time-delay dichotic conditions. *Journal of Speech and Hearing Research, 34*, 1410–1422.

Plude, D., & Doussard-Roosevelt, J. (1989). Aging, selective attention and feature integration. *Psychology and Aging, 4*, 1–7.

Porciatti, V., Fiorentini, A., Morrone, M., & Burr, D. (1999). The effects of ageing on reaction times to motion onset. *Vision Research, 39*, 2157–2164.

Pratt, J., & Bellomo, C. N. (1999). Attentional capture in younger and older adults. *Aging, Neuropsychology and Cognition, 6*, 19–31.

Pratt, J., Chasteen, A., Abrams, R. (1994). Rapid aimed limb movements: Age differences and practice effects in component submovements. *Psychology and Aging, 9*, 325–334.

Roos, M., Rice, C., & Vandervoort, A. (1997). Age-related changes in motor unit function. *Muscle and Nerve, 20*, 679–690.

Rousseau, C., & Nunes, P. F. (2002). *Home healthcare electronics: Are we ready, willing and able?* Cambridge, MA: Accenture: Institute for Strategic Change.

Rubin, G., Roche, K., Prasada-Rao, P., & Fried, L. (1994). Visual impairment and disability in older adults. *Optometry and Vision Science, 71*, 750—760.

Rumsey, K. (1993). Redefining the optometric examination: Addressing the vision needs of older adults. *Optometry and Vision Science, 35,* 363–366.

Ryals, B., & Westbrook, E. (1988). Ganglion cell and hair cell loss in *Coturnix* quail associated with aging. *Hearing Research, 36,* 1–8.

Sathian, K., Zangaladze, A., Green, J., Vitek, J., & DeLong, M. R. (1997). Tactile spatial acuity and roughness discrimination: Impairments due to aging and Parkinson's disease. *Neurology, 49,* 168–177.

Schieber, F., & Kline, D. (1994). Age differences in the legibility of symbol highway signs as a function of luminance and glare level: A preliminary report. *Proceedings of the Human Factors and Ergonomics Society, 1,* 133–136.

Schneider, B., & Pichora-Fuller, M. (2000). Implications of perceptual processing for cognitive aging research. In F. I. M. Craik & T. A. Salthouse (Eds.), *The handbook of aging and cognition* (2nd ed.). New York: Lawrence Erlbaum.

Schneider, B., Speranza, F., & Pichora-Fuller, M. (1998). Age-related changes in temporal resolution: Envelope and intensity effects. *Canadian Journal of Experimental Psychology, 52,* 184–191.

Schow, R., & Goldblum, D. (1980). Collapsed ear canals in the elderly nursing home population. *Journal of Speech and Hearing Disease, 45,* 259–267.

Scialfa, C. T., Adams, E., & Giovanetto, M. (1991). Reliability of the Vistech Contrast Test System in a life-span sample. *Optometry and Vision Science, 68,* 270–274.

Scialfa, C. T., Esau, S. P., & Joffe, K. M. (1998). Age, target-distractor similarity and visual search. *Experimental Aging Research, 24,* 337–358.

Scialfa, C., Garvey, P., Tyrrell, R. A., & Leibowitz, H. (1992). Age differences in dynamic contrast thresholds. *Journal of Gerontology: Psychological Sciences, 47,* 172–175.

Scialfa, C., Guzy, L., Leibowitz, H., Garvey, P., & Tyrrell, R. (1991). Age differences in estimating vehicle velocity. *Psychology and Aging, 6,* 60–66.

Scialfa, C., Jenkins, L., Hamaluk, E., & Skaloud, P. (2000). Aging and the development of automaticity in conjunction search. *Journal of Gerontology: Psychological Sciences, 55B,* 27–46.

Scialfa, C. T., Kline, D. W., & Lyman, B. J. (1987). Age differences in target identification as a function of retinal location and noise level: Examination of the useful field of view. *Psychology and Aging, 2,* 14–19.

Scialfa, C. T., Thomas, D. M., & Joffe, K. M. (1994). Age differences in the Useful Field of View: An eye movement analysis. *Optometry and Vision Science, 71,* 736–742.

Slawinski, E., Hartel, D., & Kline, D. (1993). Self-reported hearing problems in daily life throughout adulthood. *Psychology and Aging, 8,* 552–561.

Stevens, J., & Cruz, L. (1996). Spatial acuity of touch: Ubiquitous decline with aging revealed by repeated threshold testing. *Somatosensory and Motor Research, 13,* 1–10.

Stevens, J., & Patterson, M. (1995). Dimensions of spatial acuity in the touch sense: Changes over the life span. *Somatosensory and Motor Research, 12,* 29–47.

Tun, P., & Wingfield, A. (1995). Does dividing attention become harder with age? Findings from the Divided Attention Questionnaire. *Aging and Cognition, 2,* 39–66.

Tun, P., Wingfield, A., & Stine, E. (1991). Speech processing capacity in young and older adults: A dual task study. *Psychology and Aging, 6,* 3–9.

United States Department of Defense (1989). *Human engineering design criteria for military systems, equipment and facilities (Military Standard MIL-STD-1472D).* Philadelphia, PA: Naval Forms and Publications Center.

van den Berg, T. (1995). Analysis of intraocular stray light, especially in relation to age. *Optometry & Visual Science, 72,* 52–59.

van Rooj, J., & Plomp, R. (1992). Auditive and cognitive factors in speech perception by elderly listeners: III. Additional data and final discussion. *Journal of the Acoustical Society of America, 91,* 1028–1033.

Winn, B., Whitaker, D., Elliot, D., & Phillips, N. (1994). Factors affecting light-adapted pupil size in normal human subjects. *Investigative Ophthalmology and Visual Science, 35,* 1132–1137.

3

Designing Technology Based on Cognitive Aging Principles

Christopher B. Mayhorn,
Wendy A. Rogers, and
Arthur D. Fisk

Innovative technology design promises to enhance the lives of older adults in a variety of daily life task domains. For instance, home medical devices may allow older adults to actively manage their health care, and automatic teller machines should make banking more convenient. While the potential for improving the quality of older adults' lives with technology is great, this potential may remain unrealized unless manufacturers and designers adhere to a user-centered approach to technology development. User-centered approaches focus on the needs, capabilities, and limitations of the people who will be using these devices. Optimization of interaction between older adults and new technology is dependent on designers' understanding of the abilities of older adults.

Cognitive changes that occur with age may influence task performance in several domains. Thus, knowledge of cognitive aging research is a critical means to achieving user-centered design for this particular population. While an exhaustive review of all areas of cognitive aging research is beyond the scope of this chapter, topics covered here include memory, spatial ability, attention, and text comprehension. (For comprehensive reviews of cognitive aging phenomena, see Craik & Salthouse, 2000; Park & Schwartz, 2000).

In this chapter we will first review current cognitive aging findings to identify several general cognitive principles. For each principle, we will then discuss an instance where age-related differences in technology performance might occur, and design solutions will then be suggested. In this fashion, cognitive aging research findings will be illustrated as a method to guard against limitations and capitalize on intact capabilities in the context of technology design for older adults.

AGE-RELATED MEMORY DECLINE IS NOT UNIVERSAL

Technology usage is dependent on different types of memory. Not only must an older adult remember the procedures involved in operating a device, but he or she may also be required to initiate use at specific times or simultaneously store and manipulate incoming information during use. As the next few sections illustrate, specific types of memory decline with age whereas others are spared (Smith, 2002).

WORKING MEMORY DECLINES

Working memory tasks require temporary storage and manipulation of information in memory (Baddeley & Hitch, 1974). The mental calculation required during a visit to the grocery store is an example of a working memory task because a person may mentally calculate the cost of the items being purchased by constantly updating the total for the items placed into and removed from the shopping cart. Age-related differences in working memory are well documented (Craik, 2000) and there is some evidence that suggests that working memory decrements increase with task complexity (Craik, Morris, & Gick, 1990). Several theorists have argued that capacity limitations (Craik, 1986), speed of processing limitations (Salthouse, 1991), and an inability to inhibit unwanted information (Hasher & Zacks, 1988) may underlie these age-related declines in working memory.

One instance where age-related differences in working memory might impact an older adult's interaction with technology is the recent proliferation of automated telephone voice menu systems. Older adults using telephone menu systems to inquire about their bank balances or the status of their utility bill are required to store and process the menu options while attempting to make navigational decisions. If the structure of the menu system is very broad such that a large number of options must be considered before a choice can be made, older adults may find themselves forgetting the content of the options because their working memory capacity is exceeded. Since only one option can be chosen at a time, it must be appropriate for the goals of the older adult. Thus, all options other than the desired option must be considered as unwanted information and should be inhibited. Furthermore, if age-related working memory decline is due to reduced processing speed, the speed of menu option presentation is another factor to consider when designing computerized phone menu systems.

Design solutions derived from the cognitive aging literature can be used to compensate for age-related declines in working memory, thereby increasing the usability of the telephone menu system. Reducing the number of menu options that must be considered at each level of menu hierarchy should reduce working memory demands (Reynolds, Czaja, & Sharit, 2002). Yet another solution would be to present the most commonly requested menu items first, thereby reducing the need to inhibit unwanted options. Finally, slowing the speed of menu item presentation may also result in a more usable menu system for older adults because they will be given more time to process all of the available menu options (Reynolds, Czaja, & Sharit, 2002). The relative merits of each solution should be carefully weighed in the specific context to arrive at the best solution for all users. For example, the benefits of slowed option delivery may be outweighed by the frustration of users seeking speed and efficiency of menu navigation.

SEMANTIC MEMORY REMAINS INTACT

Semantic memory refers to the store of factual information that accrues through a lifetime of learning. Remembering the meaning of a vocabulary word, knowing the location of your doctor's office, and recognizing words and symbols are all examples of semantic memory because this information was acquired through experience. Age-related differences in the organization and use of semantic information are only slight or nonexistent, thus semantic memory remains intact throughout the lifespan (Light, 1992). When new information is encountered, it is often interpreted in the context of the pre-existing knowledge base.

Use of metaphors is one mechanism that allows an individual to utilize specific prior knowledge from semantic memory to guide behavior in novel situations such as interaction with new technology (Neale & Carroll, 1997). Thus, design strategies that capitalize on the existing knowledge base of older adults may result in more usable technology because device operation is more intuitive due to its consistency with prior knowledge. One familiar application of the metaphor principle is the Windows™ computer desktop presentation where files and folders mimic how information is organized in a traditional paper-based desktop work area. Another application of the metaphor principle lies in warnings research where metaphors have been shown to increase understanding of hazard information (Bowles, Fisk, & Rogers, 2002). For instance, the benefits of wearing a seat belt become clear when the motion of an automobile seat during an accident is equated with the motion of a catapult. Because the use of metaphors can be problematic if the metaphor does not match the individual's existing knowledge base, Bowles and colleagues suggested a methodological technique where iterative collection of normative data can be used to identify successful metaphors.

Design of electronic card-catalog systems represents one instance where metaphorical mismatches might reduce device usability. Online card catalog systems are meant to fulfill the same function as traditional card catalog systems, yet older adults' incomplete understanding of the Boolean logic underlying the database search may result in reduced ability to find information (Mead, Sit, Rogers, Jamieson, & Rousseau, 2000). In effect, older adults may have preconceived expectations for how the electronic card catalog system should work and hence be confused when they discover that the system does not operate as expected. Design solutions to remedy this metaphoric mismatch might include altering the interface of the online catalog system to more closely represent the functionality of traditional card catalog systems with which today's older cohort is particularly familiar. Alternatively, technology training should be developed to explicitly inform older users of the functionality of new systems that are inconsistent with their existing knowledge base.

PROSPECTIVE MEMORY DEFICITS VARY BY TASK

While working memory and semantic memory are forms of retrospective memory or memory for past events, prospective memory refers to remembering to do things in the future. An example would be remembering to fill the gas tank on the way home from work. Event-based and time-based prospective memory tasks vary by the demands of the task characteristics (Einstein & McDaniel, 1990).

For an event-based task, an environmental cue reminds one to perform a prospective task (e.g., placing an envelope by the door as a reminder to mail a letter). In this context, cues in the environment act as mnemonic or environmental supports that increase the likelihood of remembering the prospective task. By contrast, time-based tasks lack environmental support because they have few external cues. Time-based tasks are largely self-initiated and require one to perform an action at a certain time or after a specified amount of time has elapsed (e.g., remembering to make a phone call at 4:30 PM). Age differences in prospective memory are usually much greater for time-based than event-based tasks (Park, Hertzog, Kidder, Morrell, & Mayhorn, 1997).

Task performance in the domain of medication adherence is one instance where technology might be designed to guard against the negative consequences of age-related declines in prospective memory. Personal digital assistants (PDAs) could be an effective tool for reminding older adults to take their medications; however, the success of this type of intervention will depend on several factors such as older adults' willingness to learn to use such devices and the usability of the interface. By including environmental support in the form of a reminder or cue that is specific to the task, time-based tasks can be transformed into event-based tasks. Also, because prospective memory tasks have a retrospective component (i.e., remembering what to do) and a prospective component (i.e., remembering when to do it), an effective intervention must support both (Brandimonte, Einstein, & McDaniel, 1996). Thus, older adults will be more likely to adhere to their medication regiments if the PDA includes an auditory alarm that provides an environmental cue indicating that some action needs to be taken, and a visual display that provides specific instructions concerning what needs to be done.

SPATIAL ABILITIES DECLINE WITH AGE

The term "spatial ability" refers to one's general ability to mentally manipulate images or patterns (Shepard & Metzler, 1971). Mental rotation tasks such as those involved in determining the best approach to manipulate furniture so that it may pass through a doorframe are examples of spatial abilities used in daily life. A normative decline in spatial abilities is associated with age (Salthouse, 1992).

Of particular interest here is the strong relationship between spatial abilities and older adults' computer-based task performance (Garfein, Schaie, & Willis, 1988; Kelley & Charness, 1995). Given these findings from the cognitive aging literature, older adults' task performance may suffer in tasks that require high spatial ability such as navigating through a Web site. As older adults are becoming increasingly interested in finding information on the Web (Morrell, Mayhorn, & Bennett, 2000), design solutions that compensate for age-related changes in spatial ability are necessary to ensure ease of information access. This issue is described at length in the chapters authored by Benbow and Morrell and colleagues. Increasing environmental support through the inclusion of site maps (Mead, Lamson, & Rogers, 2002) and step-by-step navigational aids (Pak, Rogers, & Fisk, 2001) may facilitate older adults' ability to navigate through Web sites because these design options encourage them to visualize Web-site architecture and track their location within the site. Tables of content and Web-site indexes remind older adults of what information is available and where it is located, thereby facilitating navigation. Such design interventions should alleviate working memory demands by removing the necessity of storing menu information in memory. Similarly, design solutions that capitalize on the semantic knowledge of older adults should also compensate for declining spatial abilities. For example, Web-site navigation is facilitated when the organizational structure or architecture of a Web site is consistent with the pre-existing expectations and knowledge of older users (Sanchez & Czaja, 2002).

AGE DIFFERENCES IN SELECTIVE
ATTENTION ARE TASK SPECIFIC

As with memory, attention is a multidimensional construct that encompasses a broad array of processes (for a review of the varieties of attention, see Parasuraman & Davies, 1984). Selective attention is the cognitive mechanism used to filter out irrelevant information thereby allowing relevant information to be processed in memory (Rogers, 2000). Reading a book in a noisy cafe illustrates one application of selective attention because one has to avoid distraction by inhibiting the irrelevant information in the rest of the cafe to process the information that is being read. Since older adults' working memory capabilities may decline due to an inability to inhibit irrelevant information, this same phenomenon may also lead to an increased likelihood of attentional distraction in older adults (McDowd & Shaw, 2000). However, this age-related deficit in selective attention may be attenuated if an older adult has previous experience interacting with target and distractor information (Clancy & Hoyer, 1994). Therefore, age differences in selective attention are task specific to the extent that semantic knowledge relevant to the task can be applied.

Driving an automobile is one task that is highly dependent on selective attention. For this reason, any distractor that prevents a driver from selectively attending to important road cues is potentially dangerous. Thus, the removal of distractors from the internal environments of automobiles is one design solution that may improve the driving performance of older drivers. Because the visual search literature indicates that older adults can utilize environmental cues to identify relevant information (Madden, 1983), another design solution is to provide such cues during driving tasks. Driving performance of older drivers on a simulator was improved by providing cues alerting them to upcoming traffic hazards associated with left-turn intersections (Staplin & Fisk, 1991). In effect, this type of intervention acts to focus attention on relevant task-related information necessary for safe driving.

Given the conflict between older adults' susceptibility to distraction and their ability to use environmental cues, the utility of including new technologies such as global positioning systems and "heads-up" displays in newer model automobiles should be evaluated. The trade-off of potentially useful yet potentially distracting task-relevant information remains an empirical question that demands further investigation.

OLDER ADULTS' READING COMPREHENSION CAN BE IMPROVED

The ability to understand written discourse such as instructional materials is another cognitive factor that is essential for learning how to use new technology. According to the situation model approach to comprehension (Van Dijk & Kintsch, 1983), readers create a mental model for the meaning of text by interpreting it in terms of what they already know (i.e., semantic memory) and drawing inferences. While semantic memory is preserved in older adults, recent evidence from the warnings literature suggests that older adults may be at a disadvantage when they have to draw inferences in novel situations where they cannot utilize their semantic knowledge (Hancock, Fisk, & Rogers, 2001).

Following the instructions necessary to use and maintain a home medical device is one instance where reading comprehension may impact older adults' use of new technology. Interactions with home medical devices such as blood glucose monitors often entail complex procedural tasks that are often not supported by readable instructions (Rogers, Myk-ityshyn, Campbell, & Fisk, 2001). Suggested design solutions for written instructions such as those presented on home medical devices include the use of large font sizes to accommodate visual deficits, simplified sentence structure, and nontechnical terminology presented at a sixth-grade reading level at maximum (Wickens & Hollands, 1999). Other useful design solutions include the use of elaborative memory strategies (Qualls, Harris, & Rogers, 2002) and the use of explicit signals that highlight the main ideas and relations in the text (Meyer, Talbot, Stubblefield, & Poon, 1998). Consistent with the work of Hancock, Fisk and Rogers (2001), procedures should be explicitly stated so that older adults do not have to rely on inferential information.

CONCLUSION

This brief review of the cognitive aging literature illustrates the critical need for technology designers to become familiar with the capabilities and limitations of older adults. As the examples listed above demonstrate, technology can be used to augment intact abilities and compensate for abilities lost due to age-related cognitive decline. However, the successful application and usability of new technology rests on a firm understanding of the principles of cognitive aging.

Perhaps one of the most important messages derived from this review is that design solutions can and should be combined due to the interactive nature of the cognitive principles. For instance, Web-site navigation design solutions used to compensate for age-related declines in spatial ability also act to reduce working memory demands and capitalize on semantic knowledge. Likewise, a PDA auditory alarm might provide the necessary prospective memory cue to improve medication adherence, but it is also an effective means of selectively focusing attention on task-relevant information. Therefore, technology should not be designed based on one cognitive principle alone but instead should be evaluated with respect to systemic cognitive function.

Smart living environments based on ubiquitous computing systems are an example of an emerging technology that promises an holistic approach to supporting the needs of older adults (Mynatt & Rogers, 2002). Unlike earlier examples that described the application of a single device to support specific problems (e.g., blood glucose monitors), ubiquitous computing offers intervention on a much larger scale to support a variety of daily activities. For this reason, smart environment designers face the daunting challenge of developing a system that operates to support systemic cognitive function by simultaneously targeting multiple cognitive aging principles.

Presently, researchers from several disciplines working on the Aware Home Project at the Georgia Institute of Technology are developing a system to prevent accidents in the kitchen (Tran & Mynatt, 2002). Suppose that an older adult is cooking when he or she is interrupted by a knock at the door. To avoid burning the food and/or a resultant house fire, a smart monitoring system must provide a prospective memory cue that reminds the person of the necessity of completing the cooking task and refocuses attention on the fact that the stove is still on. Upon returning to the stove, the older adult must remember the last step he or she completed in the recipe prior to interruption by accessing a stove-top computer interface that acts as a surrogate for storing this information in working memory. To ensure retention of instructional information and procedural knowledge on how to use the device in semantic memory, text comprehension must be supported during initial training sessions. The interface itself should be designed to ensure that information organization is consistent with semantic knowledge and that it complements spatial abilities during system navigation.

While these smart living environments are still years away from widespread commercial use, they offer a tantalizing glimpse of the future by demonstrating the strength of multidisciplinary design that addresses cognitive aging principles. Because older adults commonly express the desire to retain their functional independence (Willis, 1996), it is clear that one approach to assist them in achieving this goal is through the development of technology tailored to meet their specific needs. It is our hope that this review provides a useful theoretical reference to guide the design of new and emerging technologies that will promote successful aging, improved safety, and personal empowerment.

ACKNOWLEDGMENTS

Christopher B. Mayhorn is Assistant Professor of Psychology, North Carolina State University. Wendy A. Rogers is Professor, Engineering and Experimental Psychology Programs, School of Psychology, Georgia Institute of Technology. Arthur D. Fisk is Professor and Coordinator of the Engineering Psychology Program, School of Psychology, Georgia Institute of Technology.

The second and third authors were supported in part by a grant from the National Institutes of Health (National Institute on Aging) Grant P01 AG17211 under the auspices of the Center for Research and Education on Aging and Technology Enhancement (CREATE).

Correspondence concerning this chapter should be addressed to Christopher B. Mayhorn, Department of Psychology, 640 Poe Hall, Campus Box 7801, Raleigh, NC 27695–7801. Electronic mail: chris_mayhorn@ncsu.edu.

REFERENCES

Baddeley, A. D., & Hitch, G. J. (1974). Working memory. In G. H. Bower (Ed.), *The psychology of learning and motivation* (Vol. 8). New York: Academic Press.

Bowles, C. T., Fisk, A. D., & Rogers, W. A. (2002). Inference and the use of similes and metaphors in warnings. *Proceedings of the Human Factors and Ergonomics Society 46th Annual Meeting.* Santa Monica, California.

Brandimonte, M., Einstein, G. O., & McDaniel, M. A. (1996). *Prospective memory: Theory and applications.* Mahwah, NJ: Lawrence Erlbaum Associates.

Clancy, S. M., & Hoyer, W. J. (1994). Age and skill in visual search. *Developmental Psychology, 30,* 545–552.

Craik, F. I. M. (1986). A functional account of age differences in memory. In F. Klix & H. Hagendorf (Eds.), *Human memory and cognitive capabilities: Mechanisms and performances.* Amsterdam: Elsevier.

Craik, F. I. M. (2000). Age-related changes in human memory. In D. C. Park & N. Schwartz (Eds.), *Cognitive aging: A primer.* Philadelphia, PA: Taylor and Francis.

Craik, F. I. M., Morris, R. G., & Gick, M. L. (1990). Adult age differences in working memory. In G. Vallar, & T. Shallice (Eds.), *Neuropsychological impairments of short-term memory.* Cambridge, England: Cambridge University Press.

Craik, F. I. M., & Salthouse, T. A. (2000). *The handbook of aging and cognition (2nd ed.).* Mahwah, NJ: Lawrence Erlbaum Associates.

Einstein, G. O., & McDaniel, M. A. (1990). Normal aging and prospective memory. *Journal of Experimental Psychology: Memory, Learning, and Cognition, 16,* 717–726.

Garfein, A. J., Schaie, K. W., & Willis, S. L. (1988). Microcomputer proficiency in later-middle-aged and older adults: Teaching old dogs new tricks. *Social Behavior, 3(2),* 131–148.

Hancock, H. E., Fisk, A. D., & Rogers, W. A. (2001). Comprehension of explicit and implicit warning information in young and older adults. *Proceedings of the Human Factors and Ergonomics Society 45th Annual Meeting.* Santa Monica, California.

Hasher, L., & Zacks, R. T. (1988). Working memory, comprehension, and aging: A review and a new view. In G. H. Bower (Ed.), *The psychology of learning and motivation (Vol. 2)*. San Diego, CA: Academic Press.

Kelley, C. L., & Charness, N. (1995). Issues in training older adults to use computers. *Behaviour and Information Technology, 14(2)*, 107–120.

Light, L. L. (1992). The organization of memory in old age. In F. I. M. Craik & T. A. Salthouse (Eds.), *The handbook of aging and cognition*. Mahwah, NJ: Lawrence Erlbaum Associates.

Madden, D. J. (1983). Aging and distraction by highly familiar stimuli during visual search. *Developmental Psychology, 19*, 499–505.

McDowd, J. M., & Shaw, R. J. (2000). Attention and aging: A functional perspective. In F. I. M. Craik & T. A. Salthouse (Eds.), *The handbook of aging and cognition (2nd ed.)*. Mahwah, NJ: Lawrence Erlbaum Associates.

Mead, S. E., Lamson, N., & Rogers, W. A. (2002). Human factors guidelines for web site usability: Health-oriented web sites for older adults. In R. W. Morrell (Ed.), *Older adults, health information, and the world wide web*. Mahwah, NJ: Lawrence Erlbaum Associates.

Mead, S. E., Sit, R. A., Rogers, W. A., Jamieson, B. A, & Rousseau, G. K. (2000). Influences of general computer experience and age on library database search performance. *Behaviour and Information Technology, 19*, 107–123.

Meyer, B. J. F., Talbot, A., Stubblefield, R. A., & Poon, L. W. (1998). Interests and strategies of young and old readers differentially interact with characteristics of texts. *Educational Gerontology, 24*, 747–771.

Morrell, R. W., Mayhorn, C. B., & Bennett, J. (2000). World Wide Web use in middle-aged and older adults. *Human Factors, 42(2)*, 175–182.

Mynatt, E. D., & Rogers, W. A. (2002). Developing technology to support the functional independence of older adults. *Ageing International, 27*, 24–41.

Neale, D. C., & Carroll, J. M. (1997). The role of metaphors in user interface design. In M. Helander, T. K. Landauer, T. K., & P. V. Prabhu, (Eds.), *Handbook of human-computer interaction*. Amsterdam, Netherlands: Elsevier.

Pak, R., Rogers, W. A., & Fisk, A. D. (2001). A further examination of the influence of spatial abilities on computer task performance in younger and older adults. *Proceedings of the Human Factors and Ergonomics Society 45th Annual Meeting*. Santa Monica, California.

Parasuraman, R., & Davies, D. R. (1984). *Varieties of attention*. San Diego, CA: Academic Press.

Park, D. C., Hertzog, C., Kidder, D. P., Morrell, R. W., & Mayhorn, C. B. (1997). The effect of age on event-based and time-based prospective memory. *Psychology and Aging, 12(2)*, 314–327.

Park, D. C., & Schwartz, N. (2000). *Cognitive aging: A primer*. Philadelphia, PA: Taylor and Francis.

Qualls, C. D., Harris, J. L., & Rogers, W. A. (2002). Cognitive-linguistic aging: Considerations for home health care environments. In W. A. Rogers & A. D.

Fisk (Eds.), *Human factors interventions for the health care of older adults*. Mahwah, NJ: Lawrence Erlbaum Associates.

Reynolds, C., Czaja, S. J., & Sharit, J. (2002). Age and perceptions of usability on telephone menu systems. *Proceedings of the Human Factors and Ergonomics Society 46th Annual Meeting*. Santa Monica, California.

Rogers, W. A. (2000). Attention and aging. In D. C. Park & N. Schwartz (Eds.), *Cognitive aging: A primer.* Philadelphia, PA: Taylor and Francis.

Rogers, W. A., Mykityshyn, A. L., Campbell, R. H., & Fisk, A. D. (2001). Only three easy steps? User-centered design of a simple medical device. *Ergonomics in Design, 9*, 6–14.

Salthouse, T. A. (1991). *Theoretical perspectives on cognitive aging*. Hillsdale, NJ: Lawrence Erlbaum Associates.

Salthouse, T. A. (1992). Reasoning and spatial abilities. In F. I. M. Craik & T. A. Salthouse (Eds.), *The handbook of aging and cognition*. Mahwah, NJ: Lawrence Erlbaum Associates.

Sanchez, J., & Czaja, S. J. (2002). The impact of organizational structure and labels on web usability for older adults. *Proceedings of the Human Factors and Ergonomics Society 46th Annual Meeting*. Santa Monica, Calfornia.

Shepard, R. N., & Metzler, J. (1971). Mental rotation of three-dimensional objects. *Science, 171*, 701–703.

Smith, A. D. (2002). Consideration of memory functioning in health care intervention with older adults. In W. A. Rogers & A. D. Fisk (Eds.), *Human factors interventions for the health care of older adults*. Mahwah, NJ: Lawrence Erlbaum Associates.

Staplin, L., & Fisk, A. D. (1991). A cognitive engineering approach to improving signalized left turn intersections. *Human Factors, 33(5)*, 559–571.

Tran, Q. T., & Mynatt, E. D. (2002). What was I cooking? Towards déjà vu display of everyday memory. *Extended Abstracts of the ACM Conference on Human Factors in Computing Systems*.

Van Dijk, T., & Kintsch, W. (1983). *Strategies of discourse comprehension*. New York: Academic Press.

Wickens, C. D., & Hollands, J. G. (1999). *Engineering psychology and human performance* (3rd ed.). Upper Saddle River, NJ: Prentice Hall.

Willis, S. L. (1996). Everyday problem solving. In J. E. Birren & K. W. Schaie (Eds.), *Handbook of the psychology of aging* (4th ed.). San Diego: Academic Press.

4

Aging and Technology—
Social Science Approaches

Heidrun Mollenkopf

AGING AND TECHNOLOGY IN MODERN SOCIETIES

A salient characteristic of most modern societies is the high degree to which technology pervades daily life. This pertains not only to the domain of industrial manufacturing and the organization of work (i.e., the reliance on information and the rationalization of services and interactions between producers and consumers), but also to the private, everyday world in which each member of society lives. Scarcely an area of human life, including the most intimate relations, is not permeated, regulated, controlled, or mediated by technology. Today several domains would in many respects be impossible without technology. Communication, mobility, keeping house, and leisure time are no longer conceivable in western industrialized societies without significant technological support. This increased use of technology opens an array of ever new alternatives for action, but it can also lead to new dependencies and unintended consequences, including alienation from other people and from direct experience, that is, the mechanization, standardization, and institutionalization of social action.

The meaning that technology's progressive infiltration of the environment has for older adults hardly needs to be emphasized in this context. An aging person's daily life and participation in society are facilitated or complicated by household technology, residential infrastructure, public and private transportation, telephones, fax machines, computers, electronic media, rehabilitation aids, and the increasing automation of services, and they depend on the design, ease of handling, proliferation, and accessibility of all these things.

Beyond concerns of everyday relevance, society in general—and the aging population in particular—are confronted by far more encompassing changes that coincide with processes of technology's proliferation. For example, during the first phases of radical change and transformation, almost every type of mechanization has led to unemployment and poverty, social inequality and disruption, and dislocation of workers and their families. Just as new social inequalities can result from different socio-structural conditions, so also can they result from technological surges, which are experienced by generations in different phases and situations of life. For instance, modern industrialized societies place great stock in the competence, performance, and output of individuals. Hence, older employees who are unable to keep pace with newly introduced technologies are often given early retirement. Worse, others are given early retirement based on the fallacious assumption that all older employees are unable to keep up with technology changes.

Increased life expectancy, due in large part to technological developments in domains as different as medical care, work life, and the private sphere of hygiene, also has a profound impact on modern lives. The emergence of old age as a separate phase of life lasting 20 to 30 years is therefore a typical phenomenon of modern industrialized economic structures. This new social phenomenon includes a great heterogeneity of individual life courses and living conditions. The differentiation of distinct, independent areas of life which emerged in the modernization processes, the individualization of values and orientations, and the pluralization of ways of life in modern society lead to an increasing diversity of individual biographies which differentiate even more strongly over time.

Communication and/or mobility become increasingly important under these conditions. If physical or sensory impairments arise, an autonomous, active life and participation in society can be seriously threatened, as dealing with the everyday world becomes more demanding. In this respect, technologies ranging from everyday appliances to complex technological systems are appropriate instruments to preserve the independence and integration of aging people.

This aspect of modernization has as yet been given little attention in theoretical discussion. Research interest in the topic tends to be problem centered, usually relating to specific areas of technology, and the nature of its treatment in empirical studies has been more practical than theoretical (Kruse, 1992). The development and use of technical aids, for instance, is being studied largely with an eye to reducing costs by replacing hospitalization with outpatient care. Other major subjects of inquiry are home adaptations and the use of technical aids from simple low-tech devices to smart-home technologies designed to help elderly people run their homes independently (e.g., Regnier & Pynoos, 1987; van Berlo, 2002); the accessibility of the dwelling's immediate vicinity, means of transportation, and the infrastructure as a whole (e.g., Owsley, 2002; Schaie & Pietrucha, 2000; Tacken, Marcellini, Mollenkopf, & Ruoppila, 1999); and the use of computers and "new media" (e.g., Czaja, 1996; Fisk & Rogers, 2002).

Recently, focus has been on user-friendly technological design, especially related to the competencies, ergonomic context, and needs of old people, and on the acceptance and use of modern technologies and integrated systems (Fozard, Rietsema, Bouma, & Graafmans, 2000; Rogers, Meyer, Walker, & Fisk, 1998; Rudinger, 1996). In particular, human factors research and gerontechnology approaches (e.g., Charness & Bosman, 1990; Fozard, 1997; Graafmans, Taipale, & Charness, 1998; Harrington & Harrington, 2000) have provided extensive, empirically based, in-depth knowledge of human-machine interactions.

However, as important as these micro-level approaches are, they often neglect the macro conditions of the complex interaction of aging and technology in modern societies' changing social and technical contexts. Clearly, they should be embedded in a more comprehensive theoretical view. Our next section shall turn to a discussion of various theoretical positions which may be useful in better integrating technology into a holistic, systems approach.

THEORETICAL APPROACHES

Issues of aging in highly technological societies can be addressed from several theoretical perspectives. Rarely are these perspectives considered jointly. On the one side are humans as social beings that naturally tend toward and depend on interaction with other humans and whose behavior, attitudes, abilities, personal relations, and forms of social organization are therefore at the center of social science research. On the other side is technology as an impersonal and neutral "entity," an artifact built by engineers and thus relegated to the purview of the natural sciences.

In between is the study of individuals and technology as studied in human factors research. Yet, this specialty has only recently begun to focus on issues of older adults. The most important integral strands of theory relevant to the subject of aging in highly technological society are summarized in the following section.

Gerontological theory offers a set of approaches that could be used to assess the impact of the spread of technology upon life in old age. Gerontological research was long dominated by the conception of old age as a decline in abilities, loss of competence, and withdrawal into passivity (Cumming & Henry, 1961). In this *disengagement* approach, a major prerequisite for successful adjustment to biological, psychological, and socially conditioned changes in old age was a voluntary and mutual loosening of, or withdrawal from, relations between elderly people and their social and spatial environment.

In the early 1960s and 1970s, this theoretical tradition came under increasing criticism as a more positive view of old age took shape. In developmental psychology it was supplanted by the concept of *life-span development* (Baltes & Brim, 1984) and in gerontology by *activity theory* (Thomae, 1983; Lehr, 2000). The former concept holds that developmental processes continue throughout a person's life span. Advanced age offers opportunities for continued growth and development if the aging person remains active and the situational conditions are favorable. Activity theory emphasizes the interaction between biological processes of aging, individual activity, and a stimulating setting. Unlike the disengagement approach, activity theory holds that the scope of activity in old age narrows only when aged persons are forced to reign themselves in because of social norms, health disabilities, or the death of family and friends.

While the positive image of aging with its emphasis on activity and physical, social, and material competence, seems preferable to forced disengagement, this picture distorts reality and can do great harm to older adults in another way. For the aged person who does not fit this ideal prototype of aging such overly positive generalizations can become a strain and even a hazard if they lead to withholding in cases where it might actually be necessary. In the course of aging most individuals will probably suffer the loss of loved ones, status, and social roles as well as increasing impairment of mobility, sight, hearing, or reactions. These changes often compromise elderly people's opportunities for autonomous living and social participation. And, in the terminology of Lawton and Nahemow (1973), environmental demands that greatly exceed an individual's competencies often yield negative affect and mal-adaptive behaviors. So, a gilded picture of old age becomes especially problematic for people suffering from an accumulation of hardships such as living alone with little social contact, major deterioration of health, low income, and poor housing. Their social situation can deteriorate further if the over generalized positive image of old age winds up serving as a political justification for reducing social services and retirement benefits.

Concepts that explicitly consider personal factors as well as conditions of the material and social environment therefore appear to be more appropriate for grasping what it means to cope with life in old age. This leads us to the discussion of theories from environmental psychology and gerontology.

Theoretical approaches in *environmental psychology* and gerontology are somewhat more promising in their ability to integrate the impact of technology into their theoretical positions by centering on human beings in their symbolically shaped and mediated environment. Environmental gerontology, in particular, focuses on the alternatives of action and experience of elderly people in their social and spatial settings. These approaches provide a theoretical perspective that can integrate biological and social aspects of aging as well as spatial and technical aspects of the environment. Briefly, these approaches hold that the action of individuals always takes place in a spatial environment that can frustrate or facilitate efforts to achieve goals of action, depending on objective circumstances and subjective perception (for more detail see Kaminski, 1976; Kruse, Graumann, & Lantermann, 1990).

According to *environmental gerontology models*, the aging organism and its capacity for adaptation are vulnerable to environmental over demands ("press") as well as under demands (Lawton & Nahemow, 1973). Generally speaking, competence in old age encompasses functions, attitudes, goals, and behaviors that are required in order to lead an autonomous, psychologically satisfying life. Accordingly, competence means that a person's ability flexibly utilizes personal and environmental resources in order to deal successfully with salient life situations and environmental demands. The specific situational and environmental conditions can foster or obstruct effective action (Kruse, 1992; Lawton, 1989).

When physical strength wanes with increasing age and a person's action radius shrinks, environmental features take on ever greater significance; misfits between behavioral competence, personal needs, and environmental conditions might undermine life quality (Carp & Carp, 1984). For instance, environmental factors such as residential situation and traffic conditions can prevent or encourage an elderly person's activities, depending on their nature. Ultimately, potential functional disabilities have far less impact under favorable conditions and with appropriate technological products than under conditions that restrict the living space of elderly people and fail to meet their needs.

Research has been limited thus far in evaluating which forms of competence and which features of the social and ecological context, and which combinations of the two, prove most effective for the psychological health and personal development of aging people. Insights into this question would be very important to the effort to shape the aging process in a way that enables people to optimally interact with their natural, social, built, and technical environments. Theoretical approaches addressing this issue could also broaden the acceptance and use of technical aids for overcoming difficult situations and optimizing environmental conditions as a person's own resources dwindle.

The relevance of biographical experiences, socio-structural conditions, and the person's own attitudes about technology were confirmed, for example, through findings of a recent German study (Mollenkopf, Meyer, Schulze, Wurm, & Friesdorf, 2000). Besides aspects of social structure such as age, household composition, income, and parenthood, attitudes towards technology were significant predictors for older adults' ownership and use of domestic appliances and modern information and communications technologies. In the latter domain, a high level of education and prior experience with technology turned out to be additional significant predictors (Mollenkopf & Kaspar, 2002).

In general, however, the trend in gerontological approaches has been to consider the aging of the human being and the attendant changes separately from the facilitating or complicating role that technology can play in this process as part of the elderly person's environment. Social integration and independent living of elderly people is not only made difficult through the loss of function of the senses or age related illness, but also through the aforementioned societal processes of differentiation and pluralization and the increasing pace of technological change.

Social science technology approaches, which could bridge the "two cultures" (Snow, 1993), because of their genuine focus on the close interaction between technology and society, have been long confined to the study of technology as an exogenous factor of change in the process and organization of work and to the theoretical treatment of technology as artifacts that either rationalize human action or give it new latitude (see, for example, Joerges, 1988). The discussion of the process of technology's pervasion of private daily life and of the concomitant changes was initially framed by the scientific paradigm of *technological determinism.* According to this view, technology constitutes a new type of rational cultural system becoming dominant in the life world of industrialized society (Ellul, 1954). All social domains of modern societies are undergoing a profound change because of an inherent logic of technology (Ogburn, 1972). Structures of thought stemming from technical subject areas are spreading more and more into originally nontechnical areas of consciousness as well—language and behavior as a whole. Consequently, the individual has no choice but to take part in technology's infiltration. The automatic nature and all-encompassing universality of that process is inescapable (Ellul, 1954).

Beginning in the mid-1970s, an opposing view of *technology as a social construct* increasingly emerged. It was no longer held that technology permeates and changes human actions with its own rationale, but that humans develop, shape, and use technology according to their abilities and interests (Bijker, Hughes, & Pinch, 1987). Since then, the theoretically conceived antithesis between being forced to adapt to technology and having the freedom to shape it, between tendencies that level out differences and tendencies that polarize, and between signs of rationalization and signs of cultivation (or recultivation) have worn down to a synthesis of both perspectives.

The aversion to separating technical, social, economic, and political aspects of technological development is illustrated in the metaphor of the *seamless web* that the social context and technology form together (Hughes, 1986). In this socio-constructivist perspective, technology is seen as a product of social processes in the course of which the social environment influences the process by which technological artifacts are created. As Bijker and Law (1992) postulated, "*All* technologies are shaped by and mirror the complex trade-offs that make up our societies . . . They reproduce and embody the complex interplay of professional, technical, economic, and political factors" (pp. 3 and 19). Conversely, they also infer that society is constructed by technology. This approach suspends the polarity represented by the "technical" and the "social."

Whether technical changes involve individual artifacts or large technical systems, the assertion that individuals or collectives generate them now seems almost trivial. The view that the environment in which people live today is much more stamped by technology than it was just 50 years ago is no doubt similarly undisputed. So is the idea that the increased use of technology is also affecting social competencies and behavior in very different spheres of life. The two views of technology are not mutually exclusive. Instead, they express different aspects of the same phenomenon. For that reason I agree with the view of technical development as a "purposeful social process" (Ropohl, 1979; our translation). But I believe that the bases of "natural phenomena and settings, human dispositions, and social conditions" (Ropohl, 1979, p. 2; our translation) must be complemented with dimensions of already existing stocks of technical artifacts, technical structures, and technical knowledge. Not in the sense of technological determination but rather of the explicit acknowledgment and inclusion of their reality as one of the important factors conditioning individual and social action alongside—or better, amid—the diversity of other structural, environmental, or social conditions.

As such a real and important environmental condition, technology is often being ignored, although the theoretical approach of the social shaping of technology can also expand the perspective of research on technology in everyday settings. From this perspective, the users of everyday technology are an integral part of the process governing technology's increasing use, and technology can be studied together with everyday life as an interactive socio-technological process.

This view also makes it possible to communicate micro-sociological and macro-sociological perspectives, for the increased use of technological artifacts in daily life leads, by virtue of their objectified problem-solving capacity, to unintended consequences for action. The rationally grounded integration of technological artifacts in daily patterns of action can give rise to new routines that open new latitude for action. Companies, institutions, and individuals find technological developments to be useful and time and energy saving, and so they acquire and use them. At the same time, the continual escalation of technology's dissemination can create new constraints and dependencies. According to the technology-spiral model developed by Braun (1993), the fact that new technology is actually used, and that it spreads, perpetuates new technological development and broadens infrastructure systems, standardization, and institutionalization of social action.

As for the daily life of older adults, the progressively wider use of technology in modern industrialized societies consequently means increasing breadth in the freedom of action and problem-solving alternatives in everyday practice. But the structuring, standardization, and anonymization of action sequences that accompany people's greater use of these alternatives are precisely what also restrict their self-determined action and direct experience. For instance, supportive infrastructure such as social service agencies and the legally mandated regulation of insurance benefits are becoming increasingly important in old age (e.g., for the provision of technical aids). The need for product standardization, the automation of services, and the increase in motorized traffic are further examples illustrating that technical developments contain both the possibilities to expand one's scope of action and to perpetuate new dependencies and limitations.

Thus, a study on the processes at work in technology's pervasion of society must consider both the specific utility that each technological artifact has for its user's objectives and the specific forms of social organization implied by its use. The effect of everyday technology can be described only in the complex micro-macro context defined by the specific patterns of individual ways of organizing things. It can be interpreted and understood only in terms of the interaction between those patterns and the artifacts and systems available in a specific society at a specific historical moment (Mollenkopf & Fozard, in press). For example, in studies on the impact of technology on household organization and family relations, structural variables such as the place in the family cycle, financial resources, and subjective attitudes and preferences have been found to be significant for the kind of technology with which families equip themselves and how they use it. The rationale by which technology was acquired differed vastly from one family to the next (Mollenkopf, Hampel, & Weber, 1989). For that reason, technology can be called a means to many ends. It thereby contributes to a differentiation and pluralization of life styles but also leads to an entrenchment of action patterns and the proliferation of existing inequalities.

Unfortunately, the promising socio-constructivist perspective of the social shaping of technology has scarcely been interested in the older adult's everyday technological reality. Therefore, a comprehensive theoretical approach for understanding the dynamic relationship between secular changes in society and technology, on the one hand, and human aging, on the other, is still to be developed.

BUILDING BLOCKS FOR A CONCEPTUAL FRAMEWORK FOR PERSON-ENVIRONMENT INTERACTIONS

This brief overview on some important strands of theoretical approaches relevant to the subject of aging in technological society should at least have pointed to the need of integrating micro-perspectives of individual aging processes (such as gerontology models of aging, research and application oriented human factors, and gerontechnology approaches), and macro-perspectives (such as sociological modernization theories) as well as socio-technological approaches which allow a combination of micro- and macro-perspectives. As stated by Mollenkopf & Fozard (in press) (see also Wahl & Mollenkopf, 2003), "Both, aging individuals and the technological products and systems they can or cannot use, are embedded in societal and technological modernization processes, and the dynamic aging and technology interaction does not least depend on the socio-structural and legislative conditions and the stocks of techno-logical artifacts and knowledge prevailing in a particular society and at a historical time."

Looking at technological products and their *symbolic meaning* might serve as an example of how the diverse approaches can be combined. In an ecologically oriented sociology of technology, or in environmental gerontology oriented primarily to technology, one must equally consider the symbolic content that objects, in this case technical artifacts, have as part of the environment for their owners and users. In phenomenolog-ical approaches the aspect of meaning is stressed, especially in relation to self-concept and identity (Fischer, 1979) (from an environmental gerontology viewpoint, see Scheidt & Windley, 2003). In sociological the-ories, by contrast, the social inequalities precipitated by the differentiat-ing character of things are highlighted (Bourdieu, 1988). In both tradi-tions, the dwelling, the home, constitutes the frame for the materialization of individual identity and social differentiation. Social constructions of this sort are also important when it comes to old age and technology, for certain images of age are conveyed via certain tech-nologies, and vice versa. As with all objects with which people surround themselves, technical objects are not neutral artifacts. They are always associated with symbolic meaning. Like home furnishings and attire, technical appliances convey to an actual or imaginary interlocutor a vis-ible expression of who the users are or how they would like to be seen.

There is a need for research on how technical objects acquire such power to create identity. For example, technical aids that can lighten environmental demands on elderly people with impaired strength or physical competence, are frequently rejected because their very shape evokes associations of handicap and disease, stigmatizing the user and undermining self-esteem. However, this may change for future genera-tions of older adults, who will have different experiences and attitudes than today's older cohorts, and when new electronic devices can be associated with the image of modernity and youth.

Further, there is the question of how technical objects contribute to differentiation as conceptualized by Bourdieu, who assumes that milieu-specific life styles are manifested in the home (and I presume outside the home) in its function as a "practical space of daily existence" in a "system of distinctive signs" and "classifiable forms of practice" (Bourdieu, 1988, pp. 277–278). "Taste therefore constitutes the practical operator for the transformation of things into distinct and distinctive signs, of continuous divisions into discontinuous polarities: Through it, the differences arising from the physical order of things become part of the symbolic order of significant distinctions" (Bourdieu, 1988, p. 284; our translation).

As far as the sociology of technology is concerned in this respect, it is possible to build on early approaches rooted in cultural and action theory (e.g., Hörning, 1985, Rammert, 1988). Hörning emphasized the symbolic character of technological artifacts and regarded the meanings attributed to them by their users as being an essential element of technology's spread in daily life. Rammert, too, concentrated less on the material or functional aspects of technology than on the perspectives and orientations of the people who develop and use technology. To both authors, the capacity of technical devices to be interpreted subjectively is the source of their cultural meaning as media conveying societal identity. Their hardware design and their individual, yet also generic, nature of use make them the means for expressing and further refining specific life styles. The "idiosyncratic" use of technology tends to foster a pluralization of life styles, as other authors, too, have shown while also relating them to the social structures that determine access to important personal and economic resources for the acquisition and use of technology (e.g., Mollenkopf, Hampel, & Weber, 1989).

Thus, summing up, social science technology perspectives seem to offer the most suitable framework for linking and integrating the most important micro and macro aspects of human aging and social and technological change in a larger societal and historical view. These perspectives can also act as a framework for and further stimulate research and application-oriented approaches to person-technology interactions. Such a wider view is needed in order to fully and appropriately account for the complex interchange processes between individuals and their technological environments.

ACKNOWLEDGMENTS

Heidrun Mollenkopf, PhD is affiliated with the German Centre for Research on Ageing and Department of Social and Environmental Gerontology, University of Heidelberg, Heidelberg, Germany.

REFERENCES

Baltes, P. B., & Brim, O. G. (Eds.) (1984). *Life-span development and behavior* (Vol. 6). New York: Academic Press.

Bijker, W. E., Hughes, T. P., & Pinch, T. J. (Eds.) (1987). *The social construction of technological systems: New directions in the sociology and history of technology*. Cambridge, MA: MIT Press.

Bijker, W. E., & Law, J. (Eds.). (1992). *Shaping Technology/Building Society: Studies in sociotechnical change*. Cambridge, MA and London, England: MIT Press.

Bourdieu, P. (1988). *Die feinen Unterschiede* [Distinction: A social critique of the judgment of taste]. Frankfurt: Suhrkamp. (Originally published as La distinction. Critique sociale du jugement. Paris: Les éditions de minuit, 1979).

Braun, I. (1993). *Technik-Spiralen. Vergleichende Studien zur Technik im Alltag* [Technology spirals. Comparative studies on technology in everyday life]. Berlin: Edition Sigma.

Carp, F. M., & Carp, A. (1984). A complementary/congruence model of well-being or mental health for the community elderly. In I. Altman, M. P. Lawton, & J. F. Wohlwill (Eds.), *Human behavior and environment* (Vol. 7. Elderly people and the environment). New York: Plenum Press.

Charness, N., & Bosman, E. A. (1990). Human factors and design for older adults. In J. E. Birren, & K. W. Schaie (Eds.), *Handbook of the psychology of aging* (3rd ed). New York: Academic Press.

Cumming, E., & Henry, W. E. (1961). *Growing old: The process of disengagement.* New York: Basic Books.

Czaja, S. J. (1996). Aging and the acquisition of computer skills. In W. A. Rogers, A. D. Fisk, & N. Walker (Eds.), *Aging and skilled performance: Advances in theory and application* . San Diego: Academic Press.

Ellul, J. (1954). *La technique ou l'enjeu du siècle*. Paris: Librairie Armand Colin [The Technological Society. New York: Knopf, 1964; Rev. Ed.: New York: Knopf/Vintage, 1967].

Fischer, M. (1979). Phänomenologische Analysen der Person-Umwelt-beziehung [Phenomenological analyses of person-environment relations]. In S. H. Filipp (Ed.), *Selbstkonzept-Forschung*. Stuttgart: Klett-Cotta.

Fisk, A. D., & Rogers, W. A. (2002). Psychology and aging: Enhancing the lives of an aging population. *Current directions in psychological science, 11*, 107–110.

Fozard, J. L. (1997). Aging and technology: A developmental view. In W. A. Rogers (Ed.), *Designing for an aging population: Ten years of human factors and ergonomics research* (pp. 164–166). Santa Monica, CA: Human Factors and Ergonomics Society.

Fozard, J. L., Rietsema, J., Bouma, H., & Graafmans, J. A. M. (2000). Gerontechnology: Creating enabling environments for the challenges and opportunities of aging. *Educational Gerontology, 26,* 331–344.

Graafmans, J., Taipale, V., & Charness, N. (Eds.) (1998). *Gerontechnology: A sustainable investment in the future.* Amsterdam: IOS Press.

Harrington, T. L., & Harrington, M. K. (2000). *Gerontechnology: Why and how?* Maastricht: Shaker.

Hörning, K. H. (1985). Technik und Symbol: Ein Beitrag zur Soziologie alltäglichen Technikumgangs [Technology and symbol: A contribution to the sociology of the everyday dealing with technology]. *Soziale Welt, 36*(2), 186–207.

Hughes, T. P. (1986). The seamless web: Technology, science, etcetera, etcetera. *Social Studies of Science, 16,* 281–292.

Joerges, B. (1988). *Technik im Alltag* [Technology in everyday life]. Frankfurt: Suhrkamp.

Kaminski, G. (Ed.) (1976). *Umweltpsychologie: Perspektiven, Probleme, Praxis* [Environmental psychology: Perspectives, problems, practice]. Stuttgart: Klett-Cotta.

Kruse, A. (1992). Altersfreundliche Umwelten: Der Beitrag der Technik [Age friendly environments: The contribution of technology]. In P. B. Baltes & J. Mittelstrab (Eds.), *Zukunft des Alterns und gesellschaftliche Entwicklung. Akademie der Wissenschaften zu Berlin* (Vol. 5: Forschungsbericht). Berlin: De Gruyter.

Kruse, L., Graumann, C. F., & Lantermann, E. D. (Eds.) (1990). *Ökologische Psychologie: Ein Handbuch in Schlüsselbegriffen* [Ecological psychology: A handbook of keywords]. München: Psychologie Verlags Union.

Lawton, M. P. (1989). Behavior-relevant ecological factors. In K. W. Schaie & C. Schooler (Eds.), *Social structure and aging.* Hillsdale, NY: Erlbaum.

Lawton, M. P., & Nahemow, L. (1973). Ecology and the aging process. In C. Eisdorfer & M. P. Lawton (Eds.), *The psychology of adult development and aging.* Washington, DC: American Psychological Association.

Lehr, U. M. (2000). *Psychologie des Alterns* [Psychology of Aging] (9th ed. / 1st ed., 1977). Wiebelsheim: Quelle & Meyer.

Mollenkopf, H., & Fozard, J. L. (2003). Technology and the good life: Challenges for current and future generations of aging people. In H. W. Wahl, R. Scheidt, & P. G. Windley (Eds.), *Environments, gerontology, and old age (Annual Review of Gerontology and Geriatrics, 2003).* New York: Springer Publishing.

Mollenkopf, H., & Kaspar, R. (2002). Attitudes to technology in old age as preconditions for acceptance or rejection. In A. Guerci & S. Consigliere (Eds.), *Vivere la Vecchiaia/Living in Old Age. Western world and modernization* (Vol. 2). Genova: Erga Edizioni.

Mollenkopf, H., Hampel, J., & Weber, U. (1989). Technik im familialen Alltag: Zur Analyse familienspezifischer Aneignungsmuster [Technology in the everyday world of families: An analysis of family specific patterns of appropriation]. *Zeitschrift für Soziologie* (5), 378–391.

Mollenkopf, H., Meyer, S., Schulze, E., Wurm, S., & Friesdorf, W. (2000). Technik im Haushalt zur Unterstützung einer selbstbestimmten Lebensführung im Alter. [Everyday technologies for senior households]. *Zeitschrift für Gerontologie und Geriatrie, 33*(3), 155–168.

Ogburn, W. F. (1972). Die Theorie des "Cultural Lag" [Cultural lag as theory]. In H. P. Dreitzel (Ed.), *Sozialer Wandel*. Neuwied: Luchterhand

Owsley, C. (2002). Driving mobility, older adults, and quality of life. *Gerontechnology, 1*(4), 220–230.

Rammert, W. (1988). Technisierung im Alltag: Theoriestücke für eine spezielle soziologische Perspektive [Technization in the everyday world: Theoretical approaches for a sociological perspective]. In B. Joerges (Ed.), *Technik im Alltag*. Frankfurt am Main: Suhrkamp.

Regnier, V., & Pynoos, J. (1987). *Housing the aged: Design directives and policy considerations*. New York: Elsevier.

Rogers, W. A., Meyer, B., Walker, N., & Fisk, A. D. (1998). Functional limitations to daily living tasks in the aged: A focus group analysis. *Human factors, 40*, 111–125.

Ropohl, G. (1979). *Eine Systemtheorie der Technik* [A system theory of technology]. München: Hanser.

Rudinger, G. (1996). Alter und Technik [Old age and technology]. *Zeitschrift für Gerontologie und Geriatrie, 29*(4), 246–256.

Schaie, K. W., & Pietrucha, M. (Eds.) (2000). *Mobility and transportation in the elderly*. New York: Springer Publishing.

Scheidt, R. J., & Windley, P. G. (2003). Physical environments and aging: Critical contributions of M. P. Lawton to theory and practice. New York: The Haworth Press.

Snow, C. P. (1993). *The two cultures* (2nd ed. / 1st ed., 1959). Cambridge: Cambridge University Press.

Tacken, M., Marcellini, F., Mollenkopf, H., & Ruoppila, I. (1999). *Keeping the elderly mobile. Outdoor mobility of the elderly: Problems and solutions*. (The Netherlands TRAIL Research School Conference Proceedings Series, P99/1). Delft: Delft University Press.

Thomae, H. (1970). Theory of aging and cognitive theory of personality. *Human Development, 13*, 1–16.

van Berlo, A. (2002). Smart home technology: Have older people paved the way? *Gerontechnology, 2*(1), 77–87.

Wahl, H. W., & Mollenkopf, H. (2003). Impact of everyday technology in the home environment on older adults' quality of life. In K. W. Schaie & N. Charness (Eds.), *Impact of technology on successful aging*. New York: Springer Publishing.

Section B

Computers, Older Adults, and Caregivers

5

Why Older Adults Use or Do Not Use the Internet

Roger W. Morrell,
Christopher B. Mayhorn,
and Katharina V. Echt

This chapter concentrates on the use and nonuse of the Internet by adults over the age of 60. Older adults, like people of other ages, use the Internet primarily for the benefits they can derive. These benefits greatly exceed simple communication between family and friends and basic information seeking. In this chapter we describe these benefits as well as several barriers to the use of information technology (computers and the Internet). Some of the explanations are myths while others are real, including barriers related to access, performance, and psychological issues. Each of these topics will be explored in the following sections.

WHY DO OLDER ADULTS USE THE INTERNET?

The Use of Information Technology by Older Adults

Although this chapter focuses on the use and nonuse of the Internet by the elderly, it would not be complete without a brief review of related literature on older adults' evolving use of computers. For example, findings spanning the past 15 years have consistently demonstrated that computers can be integrated easily into the lives of older adults in a variety of environments. These include various long-term care settings that serve frail older adults as well as the private residences of healthy community dwelling seniors (for an in-depth discussion of this topic, see Morrell, Dailey, Feldman, Mayhorn, Echt, et al., 2003). The most popular uses of computers reported by older adults include communicating with family and friends, seeking information via the Internet, improving work productivity, entertainment, and maintaining functional independence through various means (Morrell, Dailey, Feldman, Mayhorn, Echt, et al., 2003).

Clearly, older adults who use information technology can obtain several other benefits. Playing computer games has been shown to give older adults a more positive outlook on life and also could assist the elderly in developing a greater sense of emotional well-being and self-worth (Palmer, 1990; Peniston, 1990). Some researchers have suggested that interaction with computers may also improve the performance of activities of daily living, increase cognitive functioning, and decrease levels of depression (Bond, Wolf-Wilets, Fiedler, & Burr, 2002; McConatha, McConatha, Deaner, & Dermigny, 1995). Others have observed that computer use by older adults results in increased feelings of accomplishment, self-confidence, autonomy, competency, and self-esteem (Fuchs, 1988; Kautzmann, 1990; McConatha, McConatha, & Dermigny, 1994). In related research, computer training classes in community senior centers have increased active involvement among the older participants and stimulated community engagement and intergenerational social interactions (Chin, 1985). This finding and others suggest that computers might be instrumental in increasing social support for older adults on several levels (Alexy, 2000; Cody, Dunn, Hoppin, & Wendt, 1999; White, McConnell, Clipp, Bynum, Teague, et al., 1999), although Nahm (2003) suggests that more data is needed to substantiate this claim. Above all, the Internet can be an invaluable resource for communication and a source of information for older adults (Morrell, 2002a). This may be especially true for homebound individuals because communication online may reduce isolation by offering an important means of social interaction and mental stimulation, thus reducing isolation (Box, 2002). Furthermore, the Internet may serve as a gateway to information and services outside the home (Czaja, Guerrier, Nair, & Landauer, 1993; Kerschner & Hart, 1984), especially those individuals with restricted mobility (Furlong, 1989).

The Internet is expected to virtually transform health care by providing current and reliable health information to older patients and their caregivers (Brodie, Flournoy, Altman, Blendon, Benson, et al., 2000; Metcalf, Tanner, & Coulehan, 2001; Rogers & Fisk, 2001). Because older adults use health services more than other age groups, they can benefit the most from Internet-accessible health information; such information can act as a supplement to existing service provision and possibly as an online method to increase health literacy in older patients and their caregivers (Morrell, 2002b; Echt & Morrell, 2003). While these examples of increased information access demonstrate some of the current benefits older adult Internet users receive, emerging benefits include direct access to health care professionals via telemedicine (see Tran, this volume; Cresci, Morrell, & Echt, in press).

THE GROWTH IN INTERNET USE BY OLDER ADULTS

For the reasons outlined above, it is not surprising that the number of older adults online has expanded at an astounding rate. It was estimated in 2001 that more than half of all Americans between the ages of 10 and 55 used the Internet. However, the frequency of Internet use falls off steadily after age 55 (Adler, 2002; Pew Internet & American Life, 2002). Although adults over the age of 55 are less likely to be Internet users, it is important to note that older adults are surfing the Web with growing confidence and destroying myths about their reluctance to use information technology (Adler, 2002). Furthermore, as the baby boomers age, the rate of Internet use by elders will greatly expand. For these reasons the "digital divide" between generations of Internet users will diminish (Pew Internet & American Life, 2002).

WHAT ARE OLDER ADULTS DOING ON THE INTERNET?

At the turn of the century, older adults on average logged more time online (approximately 8.3 hours per week) and visited more Web sites than persons in younger age groups (eMarketer, 2000; Media Metrix, 2000). A survey by SeniorNet (2002b) indicated that 34% of their elderly respondents spent 20 hours or more per week online! Their primary reasons for using the Internet were to stay current with news and events and to research health information (see also Morrell, Mayhorn, & Bennett, 2002). Consistent with the goals of their peers who use the Internet, elderly nonusers also indicated that they would most like to learn how to access health information, use e-mail, and find information about personal travel (Morrell, Mayhorn, & Bennett, 2000). Older adults also spend more money online individually than their younger counterparts (eMarketer, 2000). The most common products purchased (ranked in descending order) are computer software, books, computer hardware, music and compact discs, and clothing (Greenfield Online, 1999; see also SeniorNet, 2002b). The range of products purchased online will certainly broaden over time as seniors and retailers become more familiar with its use. Additionally, one in ten older adults without personal access to the Internet said that they sometimes access the Internet from other places such as a friend or relative's home or the public library (Seniornet, 1998). It is important to note, however, that although there has been an upsurge in computer and Internet use by older adults, many still do not actively take advantage of the online opportunities available in the first decade of this "internet century."

REASONS WHY OLDER ADULTS DO NOT USE THE INTERNET

Three commonly held myths about why older adults do not use the Internet, computers, and other forms of electronic technology are that 1) they are less interested in learning how to use these technologies or have poorer attitudes toward their use than younger adults, 2) they simply cannot learn how to use these technologies, and 3) they are more anxious about computer use relative to younger adults, which ultimately leads to nonuse. Each of these myths will be dispelled in the next section of this chapter. We will also explore veridical explanations for why many older adults do not use the Internet.

OLDER ADULTS' LEVEL OF INTEREST AND ATTITUDES

It is true that, in general, older adults use information technology and electronic technology less than other age groups (U.S. Department of Commerce, 2002; see also Morrell & Park, 2003). However, few studies indicate that older individuals are less interested and more resistant to learning how to use information technology than are young adults (Czaja & Lee, 2001; Morrell, 2002a). On the contrary, older adults have been shown to be enthusiastic about learning how to use computers and especially the Internet, *when training opportunities are made available* (Czaja & Lee, 2001; see also Volz, 2000 for other types of electronic technology). In addition, most researchers have not found significant differences in attitudes toward computers among older individuals (Ansley & Erber, 1988). Indeed, most findings show that the majority of older adults have positive attitudes toward computers (Gilly & Zeithmal, 1985; Morris, 1994). Thus, the first myth is not affirmed.

CAN OLDER ADULTS LEARN HOW TO USE INFORMATION TECHNOLOGY?

It is with confidence that we say that older adults can learn how to use information technology, thus dispelling the second myth. It is clear that the young-old (age 60 to 74) and the old-old (age 75 and above) can readily acquire computer skills, navigate Web sites and maintain these skills over time (Echt, Morrell, & Park, 1998; Kelley & Charness, 1995; Mead, Batsakes, Fisk, & Mykityshyn, 1999; Morrell, Dailey, & Echt, 2000; Morrell, 2003; Morrell, Park, Mayhorn, & Kelley, 2000). This includes applications ranging from various commonly available software packages, to learning memory training techniques via CD-ROMs, to using specialized interactive software for health promotion (Ansley & Erber, 1988; Echt, Kressig, Boyette, & Lloyd, 2000; Egan & Gomez, 1985; Garfein, Schaie, & Willis, 1988; Plude & Schwartz, 1996). Some researchers have shown minimal or no age differences in the performance of computer tasks, for example with young and older adults (Hartley, Hartley, & Johnson, 1984) and with middle-aged and older adults(Garfein, Schaie, & Willis, 1988). Most studies indicate that computer training with older adults takes somewhat longer than with younger individuals because older adults make more mistakes than younger adults when learning to use computers (see Morrell, Dailey, Feldman, Mayhorn, Echt, et al., 2003).

THE EFFECTS OF ATTITUDES AND ANXIETY

Negative attitudes and high anxiety levels also do not seem to impact computer task performance in the elderly (Kelley & Charness, 1995). Instead, findings suggest that attitudes toward computers may be modified under certain conditions. Danowski and Sacks (1980) reported that attitudes toward computers were more positive after a three-week period of computer use by elderly residents of an urban retirement hotel. Jay and Willis (1992) utilized a multidimensional computer attitude scale to determine the effect of experience on attitudes toward using computers. They found that a two-week training program on desktop publishing resulted in attitude change on two attitude dimensions: computer efficacy and comfort. Zandri and Charness (1989) noted that training strategy appears to affect attitudes toward computers after 12 hours of training, and Kelley, Morrell, Park, and Mayhorn (1999) demonstrated that participants who returned to use a bulletin board system most often had the most positive attitudes toward computers. Positive attitude change, however, has not been observed after shorter training sessions or when participants performed poorly on computer tasks (Ansley & Erber, 1988; Czaja, Hammond, Blascovich, & Swede, 1989). Therefore, attitude change appears to depend upon the amount of exposure to the information, the content of the training, and the attitude measure administered (Jay & Willis, 1992; Kerschner & Chelsvig Hart, 1984). Findings have also shown that general level of anxiety does not predict computer task performance). Although Laguna and Babcock (1997) observed that older adults have higher levels of computer anxiety than younger adults, Charness and Bosman (1992) suggest that computer anxiety generally diminishes across training sessions. These findings suggest that concern about older computer users' performance on computer tasks being affected by negative attitudes and high anxiety may not be warranted. Rather, experience with computers appears to affect their attitudes and anxiety levels (Kelley & Charness, 1995; Ray & Minch, 1990). In short, having some experience with computers leads to better outcomes and better attitudes, thus dismissing the third myth (Mead, Sit, Rogers, Jamieson, & Rousseau, 2000).

BARRIERS TO USE

Now that we have dispelled several myths concerning why older adults do not use information technology, the remainder of the chapter will focus on some barriers that actually do limit older adults' ability to use technology. After describing the barriers we will suggest methods to overcome each.

ACCESS ISSUES

The primary reason that many older adults do not use the Internet is that they lack access to a computer (Morrell, Dailey, Feldman, Mayhorn, Echt, et al., 2003). Another reason is that they believe they cannot afford to buy their own computers or pay the monthly connection charges (U.S. Department of Commerce, 2002). These reasons for Internet nonuse are slowly being reduced or eliminated. In addition to falling prices for hardware and Internet connections, computer banks have appeared in senior centers, churches, fire stations, libraries, senior residential facilities, assisted living facilities, low income housing, and other environments. Computer access is free in most of these locales, and many offer Internet training opportunities as well. However, the access problem appears to remain in rural areas where public access sites remain geographically inaccessible to many older residents, particularly those lacking adequate transportation.

Broadband Availability. Another solution to increasing access to the Internet by older adults is by increasing broadband connections. This is currently well underway; the number of U.S. households with a broadband connection was expected to increase from 10% in 2001 to 25% by 2002 and older Internet users are currently the fastest growing segment of the population using broadband (Adler, 2002). High-speed broadband networks offer several advantages over slower narrowband networks: (a) it is possible to add high-quality, two-way video; (b) it provides instant access to rich multimedia content; (c) it makes communications more convenient, and supports a broad range of continuous, unobtrusive monitoring services; and (d) it allows the Internet to be accessed from anywhere at any time including wireless connections (Adler, 2002).

Accessibility of Web Sites. Most Web sites are designed by young people for use by young people. Thus, most Web sites are not designed to consider how age-related declines in vision, audition, perception, memory, comprehension, information processing, working memory, or motor dexterity might affect their use. This is despite findings consistently demonstrating that these factors affect how well older adults can use Web sites (see chapters in this volume by Benbow; Mayhorn, Rogers, & Fisk; and Scialfa, Ho, & Laberge for a more detailed discussion of these issues). The consequences of designers not considering the special needs of older adults is that most Web sites are inaccessible at some level to many of them.

It is important to note that Web-site design has improved over time. We no longer see multitudes of flashing banners or monkeys dancing across computer screens. Designs have been simplified and some advances have been made in improving accessibility to online information for older adults especially through products designed to enhance computer images such as the one developed by IBM (SeniorNet, 2002a) and software created by Eldervision.net called "TouchTown" that offers an alternative elder-friendly platform to access the Internet.

To further improve accessibility for the elderly, the National Institute on Aging (NIA) and the National Library of Medicine (NLM) began conducting the NIH Senior Health Project in 1999. One result from the project was the development of 25 guidelines, that when applied to Web site design, make the sites more accessible. The guidelines focus on methods to improve text readability and comprehensibility, as well as on improving navigation features. The guidelines have been systematically tested and the ease of navigation by older adults was shown to be readily improved when compared with navigation on original versions of the two sites (Morrell, 2003). The guidelines are available from NIA and NLM in booklet and online form by logging onto their Web sites (www.nia.nih.gov and www.nlm.nih.gov). The project also produced www.NIHSeniorHealth. gov, which serves as a model for Web site designers to mediate normal age-related declines in vision, cognition, and motor skills through design options. This Web site is unique in that it features the use of audio, animation, and video—complete with open captioning, in an elder friendly environment (see Morrell, Dailey, Feldman, Mayhorn, Echt, et al., 2003).

PERFORMANCE ISSUES

The Internet is searchable (Echt, 2002). The navigator scans, skips, and surfs through Web sites and bodies of text until desired information is found (Johnson, 1998). This unique feature may make it more difficult to use by older adults because it requires more complex cognitive processing. (For a discussion of these issues see chapters by Mayhorn and colleagues, and Scialfa and colleagues in this volume.)

Findings from research that investigated how the elderly conduct Internet searches generally demonstrate that they are less efficient on simple Internet search tasks and less successful overall for more complex Internet search tasks than younger adults. Kubeck, Miller-Albrecht, and Murphy (1999) found small performance differences between young and older adults on simple search tasks (those requiring six to nine steps). More difficult tasks, which required 13–16 steps, exhibited greater age-related performance differences. It is important to note, however, that with brief, well-designed training, novice older adults were successful in their Internet searches and had very positive reactions to their Internet experience. Similar results were obtained by Mead, Spaulding, Sit, Meyer, and Walker (1997). The older adults also were less efficient—they performed more procedures to find the required information than the younger participants in this research. Mead, Batsakes,

Fisk, and Mykityshyn (1999) demonstrated that older adults have more difficulty recovering from navigation errors than younger adults, especially when the number of Web pages, database records, or menus encountered exceeded two or three. These findings are consistent with the "complexity hypothesis" developed by Cerrella, Poon, and Williams (1980) which states that as cognitive tasks become more complex, greater age differences in performance will be observed (presumably due to age-related declines in cognition, i.e., working memory) (Morrell & Park, 1993). The overall conclusion is that older adults will have more problems conducting searches on the Internet until age-related decrements in cognition are considered in search design features.

AVAILABILITY OF TRAINING OPPORTUNITIES

Related to performance issues is the limited availability of training opportunities where older adults can learn to use the Internet. (Morrell, Park, Mayhorn, & Kelly, 2000). However, this barrier may be greatly reduced by incorporating training classes into continuing education programs within senior centers and elderly residential facilities. SeniorNet (www.seniornet.org) has offered computer training classes through its training centers across the country since 1986 and now includes classes on Internet use. A similar program is offered by Cyberseniors.org and AARP includes online courses on a variety of topics concerning information technology on their Web site. So, Internet training opportunities have increased for the elderly, but clearly more are needed especially for low-income seniors who cannot afford the currently offered classes.

PSYCHOLOGICAL ISSUES

Motivation. Morrell, Dailey, and Echt (2000) recently reported that another reason why older adults did not use the Internet was that they did not see any use for it in their daily lives. This is probably because many seniors are still unaware of the scope and quality of the resources available on the Internet. In short, if someone is unaware of the benefits of a product, he or she will not be motivated to use that product (Melenhorst, Rogers, & Caylor, 2001). The Hollywood adage "if you build it, they will come" does not necessarily apply to Web sites. Clearly, potential users must be made aware of a Web site, its content, and its benefits through advertising, marketing, and/or public relations campaigns before they will be motivated to visit the site.

e-TRUST. e-TRUST is generally defined as trust in information found on the Internet (Morrell, 2000). Many older adults do not use the Internet because they do not know how to verify that the information that they find there is current and reliable. This is an important issue because anyone can post information on any topic on the Internet. Some of the information is reliable and can be trusted. Some of it is not. Some of the information is current. Some of it is not. Therefore, to initiate or expand their use of the Internet, it is important to advise older Internet users how to verify the trustworthiness of information found online. (For excellent reviews of several rules that can assist older adults in assigning their level of e-TRUST for information encountered online see Benbow, in this volume; Morrell, 2000; and SPRY Foundation, 2002.)

CONCLUSIONS

In this chapter we have explored the reasons that older adults use or do not use the Internet. Clearly, older adults who use the Internet understand that there are many benefits to be gained. However, there are several reasons cited by older adult nonusers to explain why they do not use the Internet. Moreover, we discussed several frequently reported barriers to usage related to access, performance, and psychological issues. Perhaps the most important message to be gleaned from this chapter is that the barriers to older adults' Internet use can be overcome. For each barrier, we suggested a number of design solutions that can facilitate older adults' Internet use by minimizing the cognitive, perceptual, and motoric limitations that occur with age. We also described several community-based interventions such as increasing older adults' access to technology resources and training, at senior centers for example. When these barriers are eliminated and older adults become full participants in the electronic opportunities offered in the "Internet Century," those older adults who are included currently in the "digital divide" will be replaced with elderly individuals characterized by self-empowerment and increased independence.

ACKNOWLEDGMENTS

Roger W. Morrell is Director of Research, GeroTech Corporation, Reston, Virginia. Christopher B. Mayhorn is Assistant Professor, Department of

Psychology, North Carolina State University, Raleigh, North Carolina. Katharina V. Echt is Health Research Scientist, Rehabilitation Research & Development Center, Atlanta VA Medical Center, and Assistant Director, The Emory University Center for Health in Aging, Atlanta, Georgia.

REFERENCES

Adler, R. P. (2002). *The Age Wave Meets the Technology Wave: Broadband and Older Americans.* Paper presented at the National Press Club, Washington, D.C. June. Available at: www.seniornet.org

Alexy, E. M. (2000). Computers and caregiving: Reaching out and redesigning interventions for homebound older adults and caregivers. *Holistic Nursing Practice: 14,* 60–66.

Ansley, J., & Erber, J. T. (1988). Computer interaction: Effect on attitudes and performance in older adults. *Educational Gerontology, 14,* 107–119.

Bond, G. E., Wolf-Wilets, V., Fiedler, F., & Burr, R. L. (2002). Computer-aided cognitive training of the aged: A pilot study. *Clinical Gerontologist, 22,* 19–42.

Brodie, M., Flournoy, R., Altman, D., Blendon, R., Benson, J., & Rosenbaum, M. (2000). Health information, the Internet, and the digital divide. *Health Affairs, 19,* 255–265.

Box, T. L. (2002). A randomized controlled trail of the psychosocial impact of providing Internet training and access to adults. *Aging & Mental Health, 6,* 213.

Cerrella, J., Poon, L. W., & Williams, D. (1980). Age and the complexity hypothesis. In L. W. Poon, (Ed.), *Aging in the 1980s: Psychological Issues.* Washington, DC: American Psychological Association.

Charness, N., & Bosman, E. A. (1992). Human factors and aging. In F. I. M. Craik & T. A. Salthouse (Eds.) *Handbook of Aging and Cognition.* Hillsdale, NJ: Lawrence Erlbaum.

Chin, K. (1985). The elderly learn to compute. *Aging, 348,* 4–7.

Cody, M. J., Dunn, D., Hoppin, S., & Wendt, P. (1999). Silver surfers: Training and Evaluating Internet use among older adult learners. *Communication Education, 48,* 269–286.

Cresci, M. K., Morrell, R. W., & Echt, K. V. (in press). The convergence of health promotion and the Internet. In Nelson, R., & Ball, M. J. (Eds.), *Consumer informatics in an aging society.* New York: Springer Publishing.

Czaja, S. J., Guerrier, J. H., Nair, S. N., & Landauer, T. K. (1993). Computer communications as an aid to independence for older adults. *Behaviour and Information Technology, 12,* 197–207.

Czaja, S. J., Hammond, K., Blascovich, J. J., & Swede, H. (1989). Age-related differences in learning to use a text-editing system. *Behaviour and Information Technology, 8,* 309–319.

Czaja, S. J., & Lee, C. C. (2001). The Internet and older adults: Design challenges and opportunities. In N. Charness, D. C. Park, and B. A. Sabel, (Eds.), *Communication, technology, and aging: Opportunities and challenges for the future.* New York: Springer Publishing.

Danowski, J. A., & Sacks, W. (1980). Computer communication and the elderly. *Experimental Aging Research, 6,* 125–135.

Echt, K. V. (2002). Designing web-based health information for older adults: Visual considerations and design directives. In R. W. Morrell (Ed.), *Older adults, health information, and the World Wide Web.* Mahwah, NJ: Lawrence Erlbaum.

Echt, K. V., Kressig, R. W., Boyette, L. W., Lloyd, A. (1999). *Evaluating a computerized expert system for use by older adults.* Paper presented at 52nd Annual Meeting of The Gerontological Society of America. San Francisco, California.

Echt, K. W., & Morell, R. W. (2003). *Promoting health literacy in older adults: An overview of the promise of interactive technology.* Bethesda, MD: National Institute on Aging.

Echt, K. W., Morrell, R. W., & Park, D. C. (1998). The effects of age and training formats on basic computer skill acquisition in older adults. *Educational Gerontology, 24,* 3–25.

Egan, D. E., & Gomez, L. M. (1985). Assaying, isolating, and accommodating individual differences in learning a complex skill. *Individual Differences in Cognition, 2,* 174–217.

eMarketer (2000). *Senior Citizens to Embrace the Web.* Available at: www.emarketer.com/estats/dailyestats/demographics/20000918_seniors.html

Fuchs, B. (1988). Teaching elders to be computer-friendly. *Generations, 12,* 57.

Furlong, M. (1989). An electronic community for older adults: The SeniorNet network. *Journal of Communication, 39,* 145–153.

Garfein, A. J., Schaie, K. W., & Willis, S. L. (1988). Microcomputer proficiency in later-middle-aged and older adults: Teaching old dogs new tricks. *Social Behaviour, 3,* 131–148.

Gilly, M., & Zeithmal, V. (1985). The elderly consumer and adoption of technologies. *Journal of Consumer Research, 12,* 353–358.

Greenfield Online (2000). *Digital Consumer Series: The Surfing Seniors II Study.* Available at: www.greenfieldcentral.com

Greenfield Online (1999). *78 Per Cent of Senior Users Buy Online.* Available at: www.greenfieldcentral.com

Hartley, A. A., Hartley, J. T., & Johnson, S. A. (1984). The older adult as computer user. In P. K. Robinson, J. Livingston, & J. E. Birren (Eds.), *Aging and technological advances.* New York: Plenum.

Jay, G. M., & Willis, S. L. (1992). Influence of direct computer experience on older adults' attitudes towards computers. *Journal of Gerontology: Psychological Sciences, 47,* 250–257.

Johnson, R. R. (1998). *User-centered technology: A rhetorical theory for computers and other mundane artifacts*. Albany, NY: State University of New York Press.

Kautzmann, L. N. (1990). Introducing computers to the elderly. *Physical & Occupational Therapy in Geriatrics, 9,* 27–36.

Kelley, C. L., Morrell, R. W., Park, D. C., & Mayhorn, C. B. (1999). Predictors of electronic bulletin board system use in older adults. *Educational Gerontology, 25,* 19–35.

Kelley, C. L., & Charness, N. (1995). Issues in training older adults to use computers. *Behaviour and Information Technology, 14,* 107–120.

Kerschner, P. A., & Chelsvig Hart, K. C. (1984). The aged user and technology. In Dunkle, R. E., Haug, M. R., & Rosenberg, M. (Eds.), *Communications technology and the elderly: Issues and forecasts*. New York: Springer Publishing.

Kubeck, J. E., Miller-Albrecht, S. A., & Murphy, M. D. (1999). Finding information on the World Wide Web: Exploring older adults' exploration. *Educational Gerontology, 25,* 167–183.

Laguna, K., & Babcock, R. L. (1997). Computer anxiety in young and older adults: Implications for human-computer interactions in older populations. *Computers in Human Behavior, 13,* 317–326.

McConatha, J. T., McConatha, D., Deaner, S. L., & Dermigny, R. (1995). A computer-based intervention for the education and therapy of institutionalized older adults. *Educational Gerontology, 21,* 129–138.

McConatha, D., McConatha, J. T., & Dermigny, R. (1994). The use of interactive computer services to enhance the quality of life for long-term care residents. *Gerontologist, 34,* 553–556.

Mead, S. E., Batsakes, P., Fisk, A. D., & Mykityshyn, J. H. (1999). Application of cognitive theory to training and design solutions for age-related computer use. *International Journal of Behavioral Development, 23,* 553–573.

Mead, S. E., Sit, R. A., Rogers, W. A., Jamieson, B. A., & Rousseau, G. K. (2000). Influences of general computer experience and age on library database search performance. *Behaviour and Information Technology, 19,* 107–123.

Mead, S. E., Spaulding, V. A., Sit, R. A., Meyer, B., & Walker, N. (1997). Effects of age and training on World Wide Web navigation strategies. *Proceeding of the Human Factors and Ergonomics Society,* 152–156.

Media Metrix (2000). *Older Users Take to the Internet in Droves*. Available at: www.mediametrix.com/PressRoom/Press_Releases/04_04_00.html

Melenhorst, A. S., Rogers, W. A., & Caylor, E. C. (2001). The use of communication technologies by older adults: Exploring the benefits from the user's perspective. Proceedings of the Human Factors and Ergonomics Society 46th Annual Meeting. Santa Monica, California.

Metcalf, M., Tanner, B., & Coulehan, M. (2001). Empowered decision making: Using the Internet for health care information and beyond. *Caring, 20,* 42–44.

Morrell, R. W. (2000). *E-TRUST: Developing Trust in Online Health Information*. Available at: www.seniorthinking.com

Morrell, R. W. (2002a). *Older adults, health information, and the World Wide Web.* Mahwah, NJ: Lawrence Erlbaum Associates.

Morrell, R. W. (2002b, April). A Strategy to Improve Health Literacy in Older Adults: The NIHSeniorHealth.gov Project. Paper presented at the National Cardiovascular Health Conference 2002. Washington, D.C.

Morrell, R. W. (2003). *Testing the National Institute on Aging's Guidelines for Developing Accessible Web Sites for Older Adults.* Available at: gerotech.com

Morrell, R. W., Dailey, S. R., & Echt, K. V. (2000, November). *Older adults and online information.* Paper presented at the Annual Meeting of the Gerontological Society of America, Washington, D.C.

Morrell, R. W., Dailey, S. R., Feldman, C., Mayhorn, C. B., Echt, K. V, & Podany, K. I. (2003). *Older adults and information technology: A compendium of scientific research and Web site accessibility guidelines.* Bethesda, MD: National Institute on Aging.

Morrell, R. W., Mayhorn, C. B., & Bennett, J. (2002). Older adults online in the Internet century. In R. W. Morrell (Ed.), *Older adults, health information, and the World Wide Web.* Mahwah, NJ: Lawrence Erlbaum Associates.

Morrell, R. W., Mayhorn, C. B., & Bennett, J. (2000). A survey of World Wide Web use in middle-aged and older adults. *Human Factors, 42,* 175–182.

Morrell, R. W., Park, D. C., Mayhorn, C. B., & Kelley, C. L. (2000). The effects of age and instructional format on teaching older adults how to use ELDER-COMM: An electronic bulletin board system. *Educational Gerontology, 26,* 221–236.

Morrell, R. W., & Park, D. C. (1993). The effects of age, illustrations, and task variables on the performance of procedural assembly tasks. *Psychology and Aging, 8,* 389–399.

Nahm, E. S. (2003). *Social Support through the Internet and E-mail.* Available at: www.seniornet.org

Palmer, G. K. (1990). Proceedings from the Intermountain Leisure Symposium. Provo, UT: Brigham Young University.

Peniston, L. C. (1990). The mental, social, and emotional benefits of computers in a recreational program for senior citizens. In G. K. Palmer (Ed.), *Proceedings from the Intermountain Leisure Symposium.* Provo, UT: Brigham Young University.

Pew Internet & American Life (2002). *Baby Boomers and the Internet.* Available at: www.pewinternet.org/

Plude, D. J., & Schwartz, L. K. (1996). Compact Disc-interactive memory training with the elderly. *Educational Gerontology, 22,* 507–521.

Ray, N. M., & Minch, R. P. (1990). Computer anxiety and alienation: Toward a definitive and parsimonious measure. *Human Factors, 38,* 477–491.

Rogers, W. A., & Fisk, A. D. (Eds.) (2001). *Human factors interventions for the health care of older adults.* Mahwah, NJ: Lawrence Erlbaum.

SeniorNet (1998). *Research on Senior's Computer and Internet Usage: Report of a National Survey.* Available at: www.seniornet.org/research/

SeniorNet (2002a). IBM and SeniorNet Unlock the World Wide Web for Millions of Users. Available at: www.seniornet.org

SeniorNet (2002b). SeniorNet Survey on Internet Use, November 2002. Available at: www.seniornet.org

SPRY Foundation (2002). Evaluating Health Information. Available at: www.spry.org

U.S. Department of Commerce (2002). *A Nation Online.* Available at: www.ntia.doc.gov/ntiahome/digitaldivide/

Volz, J. (2000). Successful aging: 50. *Monitor on Psychology,* January, 24–28.

Wagner, L. S., & Wagner, T. H. (2003). The effect of age and the use of health and self-care information: Confronting the stereotype. *Gerontologist, 43,* 318–324.

White, H., McConnell, E., Clipp, E., Bynum, L., Teague, C., Navas, L., et al. (1999) Surfing the net in later life: A review of the literature and pilot study of computer use and quality of life. *Journal of Applied Gerontology, 18,* 358–378.

Zandri, E., & Charness, N. (1989). Training older and younger adults to use software. *Educational Gerontology, 15,* 615–631.

6

Increasing Access to Reliable Information on the World Wide Web: Educational Tools for Web Designers, Older Adults, and Caregivers

Ann E. Benbow

As noted in the previous chapter by Morrell and colleagues, a growing number of older adults are turning to the Internet and e-mail to find and share information on such key topics as health, retirement funds, travel, and hobbies. There are several barriers, which prevent extensive and effective use of these resources by older adults. This chapter describes how the SPRY (Setting Priorities for Retirement Years) Foundation set into motion a variety of efforts to reduce or remove some of these barriers, particularly as they relate to the acquisition and effective utilization of high-quality information about health care options. These efforts have included national conferences, printed guides, curricula, and training programs all designed to make health Web sites more accessible to older adults by promoting barrier free design of the sites and better training to older adults and their caregivers on how to use and evaluate the health information they find on the Internet. Seventy-one percent of Internet users between the ages of 50 and 64 have turned to the Internet for health information (Fox & Rainie, 2002). Unfortunately, they face several hurdles before they can find the best available information.

The first hurdle is finding Web sites (out of the millions on the Internet) with information that is exactly what they need, accurate, current, and understandable.

Web searching is a skill that requires knowledge of a vocabulary that is alien to many relatively new computer users (as are many older adults). While most browser software programs and Internet search engines have easy-to-use search boxes for key terms, they provide little guidance for what to do once the first list of search results appear on the Web searcher's screen. The searcher must learn to judge which links are to sites that are the most likely to be well-maintained, appropriate, understandable, and accurate. They must understand that many search engines provide "featured sites" that have paid a fee to be featured but aren't necessarily the best or, in the case of health care, promoting safe or effective products and treatments. Once having arrived at a promising Web site, the older adult user is faced with finding the information on the site and evaluating it for usefulness and reliability. Many Web sites compound this problem since they are not designed to be user-friendly to the older adult audience, many of whom may have deficits in the perceptual, motor, or cognitive capacities necessary for successful navigation and use. Fonts may be too small, contrast between the screen objects and background may be insufficient, buttons may be hidden, tags may be missing, menus may be confusing, colors may be too strident or too muted, and pop-ups may appear, all making the task of finding information on the site difficult or impossible.

The SPRY Foundation recognized Web site design for older adults as a serious problem as a result of its 1999 NIH conference on Older Adults, Health Information, and the World Wide Web. To address this problem, SPRY produced guidelines for Web site developers on how to design a health Web site that is user-friendly to the older adult user. The guide provided advice in such areas as:

- Font type (use sans-serif fonts such as Helvetica or Arial)
- Font size (14-point or greater)
- Scrolling (keep to a minimum; use Next and Back buttons and shorter pages instead)
- Color choice (primary colors, rather than pastels)
- Contrast (dark objects on a light background, or vice-versa)
- Buttons (large and clearly tagged so that screen readers can read them)
- Menus (top or side and clearly labeled in everyday language)

- Graphics (large, appropriate, tagged, and useful to the content of the site)
- Text amount (enough to fit on one page without too much scrolling)
- Text location (centrally placed on the page)
- Site complexity (ideal if the site is only a few mouse clicks deep)

The guide was disseminated to all members of the U.S. Congress as well as all Area Agencies on Aging in the country and is downloadable from the SPRY Web site (www.spry.org) as a PDF file.

Once the older adult user finds the desired information on a Web site, he or she must evaluate it for its accuracy, currency, and usefulness for his or her situation. With health information, in particular, this evaluation process poses an enormous problem. Since the content on the Web is unregulated, Web site sponsors can, literally, put anything on their sites they want without content specialist oversight or any penalties for misinformation. Inexperienced Web users can be easy prey for health Web sites that promise spectacular cures or give spurious health advice, often for a fee.

Fortunately, several public and private groups have recognized the enormity of this problem and have provided guidelines for consumers to help them evaluate health content on Web sites. These groups include, among others, Health on the Net (www.hon.ch), Hi-Ethics (www.hiethics.org), the British Healthcare Internet Association (www.bhia.org), and the Internet Healthcare Coalition (www.ihealth-coalition.org). They give Web site searchers guidelines to follow in evaluating health Web sites designed to help the user ascertain if the site is supported by a legitimate organization. They include:

- *Accuracy:* How do you know the information is accurate?
- *Authorship:* Do you know who developed the site's content? What are their credentials?
- *Currency:* How current is the site's information? When was it updated last?
- *Funding Source:* Who is behind the site? What interest do they have in it?
- *Copyright Ownership:* Do the sponsors own the copyright to the information on the site? If not, is the information attributed to the copyright owners?
- *Privacy Statement:* Is privacy protected while visiting the site?

- *Disclaimers:* Do the site sponsors remind you that information on the site should not take the place of consultation with a health care professional?
- *Contact Information:* Is there easy-to-find contact information on the site with names, addresses, and phone numbers?

As a result of our second NIH-sponsored conference in February 2001 on *Older Adults, Health Information, and the World Wide Web,* the SPRY Foundation recognized the need to widely disseminate to older adults and caregivers information about how to evaluate the content of health Web sites. This need was subsequently supported by the findings of the Pew Internet Study, which states:

> Experts say that Internet users should check a health site's sponsor, check the date of the information, set aside ample time for health search, and visit four to six sites. In reality, most health seekers go online without a definite research plan. The typical health seeker starts at a search site, not a medical site, and visits two to five sites during an average visit. She spends at least thirty minutes on a search. She feels reassured by advice that matches what she already knew about a condition and by statements that are repeated at more than one site. She is likely to turn away from sites that seems to be selling something or don't clearly identify the source of the information. And about one-third of health seekers who find relevant information online bring it to their doctor for a final quality check.
>
> Only about one-quarter of health seekers follow the recommended protocol on thoroughly checking the source and timeliness of information and are vigilant about verifying a site's information every time they search for health information.(Fox & Rainie, 2002, 4).

It was clear that the task was to assist seniors and their caregivers in effectively finding accurate and reputable sources on the Web by providing them with a basic protocol to follow. In anticipation of the need for such a protocol, the SPRY Foundation took two practical steps. First, we collected and analyzed a set of Web-site evaluation guidelines from several national and international health Web-site watchdog groups, e.g., Health on the Net and Hi-Ethics, looking for areas of agreement across the guidelines. SPRY then published a synthesis of the guidelines in a brochure entitled *Evaluating Health Information on the WWW: A Guide for Older Adults and Caregivers* (Benbow, 2001). This brochure, in both English and Spanish, was also disseminated to all members of Congress and to all Area Agencies on Aging across the U.S.

The second step SPRY took to support the use of a protocol in seeking health information on the Internet was to develop and test a curriculum for older adults and caregivers on finding and sharing reliable health information from the Internet. The curriculum includes the *Guide,* as well as instruction on basic e-mail use and Internet search and navigation techniques. E-mail was included as one of the easiest and most efficient ways of sharing reliable Internet health information once it is located. In collaboration with several government, and not-for-profit entities, SPRY has begun to disseminate the curriculum widely. We will next discuss the steps that were involved in this discussion process.

BACKGROUND ON THE INTERNET TRAINING COURSE FOR OLDER ADULTS AND CAREGIVERS

In 2000, SPRY was asked by the New Jersey Department of Health and Senior Services (NJDHSS) to assess the level of computer (specifically, Internet) use by Area Agency on Aging (AAA) staff in New Jersey's 23 counties. Computers had recently been installed in all the AAAs to improve quality of service to the community, and state officials wanted to ensure that staff had adequate training in e-mail use and Internet search, as well as adequate access to the new machines. Working with Rutgers University, SPRY developed and distributed a survey instrument to all AAA executive directors and staff, assessing their skill levels and access to work computers. Survey results demonstrated that, while the executive directors felt that they and their staff members had sufficient training and access to the computers, the AAA staff, mostly information and referral specialists, felt extremely unprepared. As a result of these findings, the NJDHHS asked the SPRY Foundation in 2001 to design and implement a training program in Internet use that would help their AAA staff to find the most current and reliable information on health and senior services for the older adult population of New Jersey and to communicate that information to clients. This course was designed as a master training session that would benefit the AAA staff directly, but would also be taken into the community to be used with older adults in their homes and other residential settings.

The course, eventually the basis for both an instructional video and an interactive CD-ROM, covered e-mail basics, Internet search, and content evaluation. It emphasized finding and transmitting information vital to older adults and their caregivers. Particular focus was given to accessing information on health, health care, social security, insurance, nursing homes and other specialized housing, Medicare and Medicaid, transportation assistance, and hospice services.

In 2002 and again in 2003, after the release of the Pew Internet study, the course was revised to place a stronger emphasis on using a systematic approach to Internet search for health information. An addendum to the basic course included information on advanced Web search skills (Boolean search terms, meta-search engines, Invisible Web). With funding support from the U.S. Administration on Aging, the revised basic course was used as the source material for master training of staff from state departments of aging in Arkansas, Iowa, Maryland, Nevada, and Pennsylvania.

The revised course was designed to be a model for professional caregivers to use in the community with older adults. Consequently, the instructional methods included techniques that have been found to be effective in older adult computer training (Zandri & Charness, 1989; Czaja, Hammond, Blascovich, & Swede, 1989; Morrell, Park, Mayhorn, & Kelley, 2000), such as: (a) providing a hard copy course guide, with simple, step-by-step directions, to be used as a reference throughout the course; (b) allowing ample time for practicing skills with expert help available; (c) pairing more adept students with less adept; (d) keeping class sizes small; (e) frequent review; and (f) repeated demonstrations of each technique.

Each participant received a pretest assessment of Internet knowledge and skills. Follow-up assessments were conducted one week and six months after training to determine the extent to which they used the course material with older adults in the community. The results of the assessments (administered and analyzed in 2002 by Nicholas Castle, PhD, Rand Corporation) showed that the training doubled the percent of participants who rated their e-mail skills and their Internet searching skills as "good" or "very good." Sixty-seven percent of the participants used their e-mail skills from the course to train others at work on e-mail and 81 percent on locating and searching Web sites useful to older adults.

COURSE STRUCTURE AND IMPLEMENTATION

The original New Jersey courses were taught in a 14-station computer laboratory in Trenton, equipped with a master computer projection system and T1 Internet access. Each participant had a computer and received a course guide and a floppy disk to store any information they found useful from their Internet searching. Two or more instructors were usually in the room during training. Most classes had 12 or fewer participants. While course organizers had hoped that participants in each group would have similar skill levels, some groups were quite variable in skills and required more instructional assistance and time. In these heterogeneous groups we attempted to pair a more skilled participant with one who was less skilled.

Each participant was assigned an e-mail account for use in the course and these were posted in the classroom. Each participant's computer desktop included an MS Word document, which assisted in demonstrating attachments. Training topics were generic enough to address a variety of e-mail systems. This ensured that when participants worked with older adult clients, they could address clients' specific e-mail needs. The topics included composing, receiving, opening, and forwarding messages; sending, receiving, downloading, and storing attachments; setting up address books; organizing messages into folders; e-mail etiquette; deleting unwanted e-mail; and avoiding e-mail-borne computer viruses. For each topic the instructor first discussed and demonstrated, and then participants practiced.

In the precourse survey, participants had expressed a desire to learn how to manage their e-mail for the greatest efficiency and safety. They particularly wanted to know how to set up and use an address book and organize their e-mail so that messages were easy to find later on. The instruction demonstrated how to set up and use address books for several major types of e-mail systems, but also included a warning about how some viruses can be spread via address books. Participants were then shown how to set up an e-mail folder system, including main and subfolders, and how to move their e-mail into these folders.

An important part of using e-mail, both professionally and personally, can be described as "e-mail etiquette." Participants discussed concerns about how they and colleagues used e-mail, and suggested ways to address these concerns. In providing e-mail training to their older adult clients, they particularly wanted to avoid passing on information or techniques that would result in any online abuse or other problems. They wanted to be able to help their clients share reliable health information with family and friends via e-mail, without having those clients compromised by their lack of e-mail knowledge. This discussion was blended with the course material to yield the following suggestions for e-mail etiquette:

- Do not forward an e-mail to a third party without the permission of the original sender. This is particularly important if the e-mail contains sensitive or personal information.
- Do not include information in an e-mail that you would not want to have forwarded to a third party without your permission. Such information might include social security numbers, bank account numbers, workplace gossip, credit card information, health issues, or other sensitive data.
- Make sure that an auditory signal for new e-mail on your computer does not irritate those around you. This is particularly true if you are working in an open office space, where such "pings" can be heard easily.
- Do not send jokes or other nonwork e-mail to colleagues' work e-mail systems. In most work settings, this can be seen as unprofessional and a waste of time.
- Do not copy people unnecessarily on e-mail. Every e-mail takes time to open and read. Being copied unnecessarily is a waste of time.
- Check the "cc" list before forwarding a message to a colleague. This helps to avoid duplication of effort, so that the recipient is not receiving the same message from several sources.
- Use a professional tone in work e-mail, as well as correct grammar, spelling, and pronunciation.
- When sending attachments, double check to be sure that the file is actually attached.
- Check with your recipient before sending an attached file, to ensure that he or she has the software needed to open the file.
- When sending very important e-mail, such as an online job application with attached resume, follow up with a telephone call to verify its receipt.
- Remember that, once an e-mail is sent, it can be forwarded to *anyone* else who has an e-mail account. Always read e-mail over carefully before sending, to ensure that you are comfortable with the information being transmitted.

Next, the class proceeded to learning a variety of Web-related skills, including: using search engines, accessing Web sites, evaluating promising search results, navigating around Web sites, using the site map to find information, and managing the information obtained (printing, copying, and bookmarking).

SEARCH ENGINES

Participants learned to use a search engine by keying their own names into the search window on Google (www.google.com). Google was selected as the practice search engine due to its extremely simple interface and searching power. When the initial list of citations appeared on participants' screens, they were asked to make a note in their course guides of how many citations they had. They were then invited to browse the list and explore some of the links. After a period of checking through the first list of links, participants stopped for some direct instruction on what to look for in the Web addresses. They learned about different domain types (.edu, .gov, .com, .org), and discussed the relative reliability of each, particularly with regard to health information. They then learned about constructing search strings to narrow their searches (using quotation marks, and some basic Boolean terms), then re-searched Google, again using their own names, but with additional search information. They were able to see, from the number of citations they had on the second search, the power of restricting and refining their search.

WEB SITE BASICS

Participants learned basic Web site terminology by exploring two major federal government web sites: MEDLINE plus (www.medlineplus.gov), the consumer health Web site from the National Library of Medicine; and Medicare.gov (www.medicare.gov) from the Centers for Medicare and Medicaid Services. These sites were selected for their elder-friendly design, reliability, and importance of information to the older adult audience. Participants learned to navigate these sites, but also learned about generic Web terms such as menus, buttons, site maps, hyperlinks, privacy statements, contact us, and banners.

Once participants felt comfortable browsing these sites, they were encouraged to explore other sites of value to older adults, such as the Social Security Administration (www.ssa.gov), Benefits.gov (www.govbenefits. gov), Benefits Check-up (www.benefitscheckup.org), Healthfinder, from the U.S. Department of Health and Human Services (www.healthfinder.gov), the National Institutes of Health (www.nih.gov), the National Institute on Aging (www.nia.nih.gov), the Centers for Disease Control and Prevention (www.cdc.gov), and the U.S. Administration on Aging (www.aoa.gov).

MANAGING INFORMATION FROM WEB SITES

Participants learned to capture and attribute information from Web sites using a page from MEDLINEplus describing the side effects of a medication in common use among older adults (Glucatrol—for control of diabetes). They learned how to copy and paste the text into a word document, how to print specific text vs. entire web pages (print "selection" on the print menu), how to bookmark the page for later reference, and how to paste text into e-mail messages. They also learned the importance of citing the source of this information in documents and e-mail.

EVALUATING HEALTH INFORMATION ON WEB SITES

Participants ended the training course by comparing the health information on MEDLINEplus to several health Web sites sponsored by non-profit organizations (such as the American Heart Association and the American Lung Association) and commercial entities (such as WebMD). They used the SPRY *Guide* as their source material to compare the reliability of health information on the sites from .gov, .org, and .com domains. They then shared their observations with other class members, focusing on such aspects of the information as authorship, currency, and accuracy. Many participants were surprised by the wide variation in amount and quality of health information on the same topic from site to site. They felt that this exercise was useful partly because it gave them one or two comprehensive and reliable Web sites they could regularly depend on.

SUMMARY

The number of health and benefits Web sites will only grow in coming years. SPRY's Internet education work for a variety of audiences (Web site designers, older adults, and formal and informal caregivers) has been designed to streamline the process of finding information on the Internet by improving Web site design; training professional caregivers and older adults in Internet use; and developing and disseminating a set of resources to support both the design and training efforts. The ultimate goal of the SPRY Internet programs is to improve older adults' access to the most current and reliable health and benefits information available on the Internet.

In summary, older adults' use of e-mail and the Internet is growing rapidly, particularly for finding and transmitting information about health. The number of health and benefits Web sites is also growing rapidly. While these can be viewed as positive trends, the unregulated nature of information on the Internet means that unwary users can easily fall prey to health fraud schemes or think that incorrect health information is accurate just because it is on a Web site. They can also waste considerable time searching through poorly designed and/or poorly maintained Web sites. Only through education about how to access, evaluate, and communicate information on the Internet can older adults take optimum advantage of this enormous resource. SPRY Foundation has sought to meet that educational need by developing and disseminating a design guide for Web site creators, a booklet on evaluating health information on the Internet, and a master training course in Internet use for older adults and professional caregivers in six states.

ACKNOWLEDGMENTS

Ann E. Benbow is Chief Consultant at the SPRY Foundation in Washington, D.C.

REFERENCES

Benbow, A. (2001). *Evaluating health information on the WWW: A guide for older adults and caregivers.* Seattle: Caresource Healthcare Communications.

Czaja, S. J., Hammond, K., Blascovich, J. J., & Swede, H. (1989). Age-related differences in learning to use a text-editing system. *Behaviour and Information Technology, 8,* 309–319.

Fox, S., & Rainie, L. (2002). *Vital decisions: How Internet users decide what information to trust when they or their loved ones are sick.* Washington, DC: Pew Internet & American Life Project.

Morrell, R. W., Park, D. C., Mayhorn, C. B., & Kelley, C. L. (2000). The effects of age and instructional format on teaching older adults how to use ELDERCOMM: An electronic bulletin board system. *Educational Gerontology, 26,* 221–236.

Zandri, E., & Charness, N. (1989). Training older and younger adults to use software. *Educational Gerontology, 15,* 615–631.

7

Computer-Mediated Communication and Its Use in Support Groups for Family Caregivers

Kathleen A. Smyth and Sunkyo Kwon

COMPUTER-MEDIATED COMMUNICATION FOR THE ELDERLY

Of all the technological aids discussed in this book, computer-mediated communication (CMC) is the most likely to remain essentially the same for some time to come. The quality of the communication can be expected to further improve, the characteristics of the users are likely to change (e.g., more elderly, female, and individuals of low socioeconomic status will reduce the so-called "digital divide"), and the frequency of use is likely to rise. However, CMC has natural limits because there are no conceivable alternatives to text-, audio- and video-based communication systems. In the future, the "telepresence" or "e-presence" of current CMC may be superseded by some sort of virtual-reality technology that will make distance communication appear like "real" face-to-face (FTF) communication. We place quotation marks around the word "real" in the previous sentence because, while CMC is irrefutably real, "real communication" in everyday language currently alludes to verbal interactions in close, direct, physical proximity, e.g., seeing/hearing the partner(s) at a conventional communication distance.

Microprocessor-based enhanced/enriched/augmented communication can bring us many new, qualitatively different opportunities if researchers and practitioners choose to move away from attempting to provide the closest possible parallel to "natural communication." It is conceivable that some kind of "artificial communication" could be brought into use. These topics, however, are beyond the scope of this chapter.

Regardless of the exciting technological developments the future may hold, text, audio, and/or video as distance communication devices will continue to address the social-interaction needs of the vision- and/or hearing-impaired, whose numbers are high in elderly populations. In this context, CMC or microprocessor-controlled communications are secondary media and treated as "tools" as compared with "natural" communication that is represented by traditional FTF interaction (cf., Pross, 1972). Hence, professionals in gerontological research and practice alike need to be thoroughly informed about and prepared to cope with the various shortcomings of such communication modalities.

For the foreseeable future, researchers, educators, trainers, and users involved with CMC must continue tackling the problems associated with communication that may not or does not reflect the FTF situation, including possible distortion of message content due to changes of affect, identity, and/or behavior, idiosyncrasies in group dynamics if group interaction takes place, and the like. For example, it is not fully understood whether CMC results in the same level of interpersonal understanding as FTF communication. Consider, for example, the way written and spoken communication often differ, how behavior changes when individuals are observed, and how in-person communication differs from phone communication. It is readily noticeable to the average observer that there are differences between FTF verbal communication and verbal communication by telephone, in, for example, the ways of introducing oneself to a stranger or the amount of detail provided to describe a physical object or an experience or in giving directions. There are also likely psychological differences, such as in the extent of risk-taking behavior, self-disclosure, politeness, aggression, or altruism. Special kinds of group conflicts in CMC are codetermined by the characteristics of identities that can only be formed on the Internet (Vrooman, 2002). The kind of medium selected for communication may evoke different internal and external states in individuals that may change over time.

However, there is no conclusive evidence as to whether the impacts are negligible or whether they affect our very essence or selves—our personalities, our identities, and/or our behavior. It is also important to consider that if an individual belongs to a social, cultural, political, or demographic subgroup, CMC can promote and reinforce an individual's understanding about and identity with the subgroup (McKenna & Bargh, 1998). This phenomenon might be beneficial, but it might also be harmful.

Thus, mainstreaming today's gerontologically focused CMC technology requires empirical evidence. CMC and the support and therapeutic modalities based on it are as efficient and effective as conventional/traditional ways of helping older clients. This chapter explores these issues by reviewing the theory and empirical findings associated with the design and implementation of CMC-based caregiver support groups.

CAREGIVERS AND CAREGIVING

THE WHO AND WHY OF CAREGIVING

Over eight million older adults in the U.S. need personal, social, and/or medical assistance to deal with chronic illnesses and disabilities, and the number is expected to nearly triple over the next 30 years. Most of them are able to live in the community, rather than in nursing homes, thanks to help received from family and friends. These helpers, commonly called informal caregivers (to distinguish them from professional individuals or organization that give care), provide most of the assistance ill or disabled older adults receive (Caregiving, 2000). Family caregivers have aptly been called the backbone of the long-term care system for the elderly in the U.S. Without the help they give, the country's health and social service providers would be overwhelmed by the care needs of the frail and disabled (McConnell & Riggs, 1994). While we focus here on data from the U.S., it is important to remember that the impact of the demographic trends underlying events we describe is being felt worldwide.

Often there is a "primary" caregiver, usually a family member, who takes on most or all of the responsibility for an older individual in need. Other family members and friends often provide specific types of help on a regular basis or provide help sporadically. Husbands and wives are usually first in line to become caregivers when their spouse is faced with illness or disability. However, they may often need assistance themselves, and many older adults are widowed, divorced, or have never married. Consequently, adult children, especially daughters and daughters-in-law, constitute the largest proportion of family caregivers (A Portrait of Informal Caregivers in America, 2001). Caregivers may face a wide variety of tasks ranging from meal making, shopping, housework, transportation, and bill paying to providing assistance with eating, dressing, and bathing, walking, medications, and medical devices. They must often provide supervision to ensure safety, and arrange or coordinate care provided by paid caregivers (Caregivers of Those with Alzheimer's, 1999; The Wide Circle of Caring, 2002).

This profile of caregiving and caregivers is drawn from studies of the U.S. However, it is important to note that the phenomena described are or will be experienced worldwide as we continue into the 21st century.

CAREGIVING IMPACTS AND THE ROLE OF SUPPORT GROUPS

Numerous studies have shown that caregivers often experience high levels of stress stemming from the provision of care itself coupled with the need to meet competing demands of family, job, and society. The resulting negative mental and physical health effects have been well-documented (Schulz, O'Brien, Bookwala, & Fleissner, 1995), and interventions that can ameliorate the negative impacts of caregiving and enhance caregivers' ability to maintain the caregiving role are avidly sought. Support groups are among the most frequently recommended caregiver interventions. Although evaluation studies of support group effects have yielded mixed results (Bourgeois & Schulz, 1996), there is widespread belief that support groups benefit caregivers (Gonyea, 1989). Caregiver support groups typically have 5–15 members who meet face-to-face (FTF) on a regular basis, usually once a month. Groups can be open or closed, ongoing or time limited. They are intended to provide a safe, supportive environment in which caregivers can share their experiences and learn from others; obtain needed information; acquire problem solving skills; receive encouragement to maintain their own health; experience personal growth and development; and have the opportunity to socialize with others and take a break from caregiving responsibilities (Alzheimer's Association, 1995). Some distinguish support groups lead by professionals from self-help or mutual aid groups composed of lay people who share a common problem or need (King &

Moreggi, 1998). In this chapter, the term support group is used to encompass both types of groups.

There are several drawbacks to FTF caregiver support groups: Caregivers' time, energy, and other resources tend to be severely limited, making it difficult for caregivers to find and connect with a support group on a regular basis; since FTF groups generally meet on a fixed schedule, the issues important to an individual caregiver may not be addressed in a timely way; not all caregivers feel comfortable seeking support in public settings; in rural areas, caregivers may live too far away from one another to make FTF meetings feasible; and ethno-cultural factors may keep ethnic minorities from support group participation (Henderson, Gutierrez-Mayka, Garcia, & Boyd, 1993; Schmall, 1984; Wright, Lund, Pett, & Caserta, 1987).

In the late 1980s, clinicians and researchers began developing computer-mediated caregiver support groups (CMSGs) to replace or supplement FTF groups. The remaining sections of this chapter give a rationale for these attempts, describe several exemplars, summarize pertinent research findings, and identify computer-mediated support group (CMSG) strengths and weaknesses, discuss their practice implications, and identify future research needs.

THE EMERGENCE OF
COMPUTER-MEDIATED SUPPORT GROUPS

RATIONALE

In the mid-1980s, Rogers (1986) and others began describing the characteristics of computer-mediated communication (CMC) systems, and interventionists soon began to see the potential suitability of CMC systems for implementing caregiver support groups. One clear advantage was that with CMC systems, many individuals can be reached simultaneously (as in mass communication), yet individual needs can be articulated and responded to as well (as in interpersonal communication) (Rogers, 1986). Another advantage was that CMC can be asynchronous—the sender and receiver of a message do not have to be available to communicate at the same time. These essential features of CMC made CMSGs appear feasible.

CMSGs have proliferated. Entering the phrase "caregiver online support groups" into an Internet search engine will yield thousands of links.

Unfortunately, most CMSGs have not been evaluated. This chapter features a selected group of CMSGs about which evaluative information has been published in the peer-reviewed literature or presented at professional meetings.

Exemplars

CMSG developers face many choices: Will the group be open to all or limited to a certain target group? Will the group be ongoing, or will it end at a pre-established time? What technology will be used for implementation? Will the CMSG be integrated with other caregiver information and support services, or will it stand alone? Will the group have a moderator, or will it be entirely run by caregivers themselves? If a moderator is identified, what role(s) will s/he play? What type of registration process, if any, will be required?

Tables 7.1 and 7.2 give descriptive information on seven CMSGs designed to support family caregivers sampled from the research or clinical literature; collectively, they illustrate various combinations of answers to the key questions posed above. One CMSG listed is not identified by name in the article describing it. This decision reflects one of several conflicting views on the norms that should govern research on the Internet. (See Frankel & Siang, 1999, for an overview of key issues.) Tables 7.1and 7.2 are followed by some additional information on the selected groups.

Although several of the CMSGs listed in Table 7.1 are embedded in systems with additional features, this chapter focuses on their attempts to facilitate caregiver-to-caregiver interaction. While each of the CMSGs is moderated, the approaches reflect several possible roles the moderator might take (Berge, 1994). These include facilitator/group leader; manager/administrator; filter (controlling postings); expert; editor; discussion promoter; marketer; general helper; and firefighter (preventing "flames" or ad hominem attacks). Each group involves some level of promotion, marketing, and management. The Alzheimer's Disease Support Center (ADSC), The Alzheimer List, and the group for mental health caregivers have less intense facilitator involvement than the other groups, which involve protocol-driven monitoring by professionals.

Each of the exemplars has undergone some type of systematic evaluation. The following section summarizes what has been learned from these and other studies.

TABLE 7.1a Computer-Mediated Support Group Exemplars: Sponsorship, Focus, and Technology Used

Project, Sponsor, Funding and Key Reference	Focus	Technology Used
Alzheimer's Disease Support Center (ADSC), University Hospitals of Cleveland/Case Western Reserve University, Cleveland OH; Funding: National Institute on Aging Alzheimer's Disease Center Grant (Smyth, Feinstein, & Kacerek, 1997)	Alzheimer's disease and related conditions	Originally text-based Internet site but now Web based, accessed by personal computer
Caring-Web©, Medical College of Ohio, Toledo, OH; Funding: Maumee Bay Chapter, Assoc. of Rehabilitation Nurses, Zeta Theta and Nu Delta Chapters, Sigma Theta Tau International, Medical College of Ohio, and Cleveland State University (Pierce, Steiner, & Govoni, 2002)	Stroke	Web based, accessed by WebTV© or personal computer
ComputerLink, Case Western Reserve University, Cleveland OH; Funding: National Institute on Aging R01 grant (Brennan, Moore, & Smyth, 1995)	Alzheimer's disease and related conditions	Text-based Internet site accessed by terminals
Link2Care, Family Caregiving Alliance, San Francisco, CA; Funding: California Dept. of Mental Health purchase of service dollars (Kelly, Johnson, & Eskenazi, 2001)	Alzheimer's disease and related conditions	Web based, accessed by personal computer
REACH for TLC (Telephone Linked Care), Hebrew Rehabilitation Center for Aged, Boston, MA; Funding: National Institute on Aging REACH multi-site collaborative project (Mahoney, Tarlow, & Jones, 2003)	Alzheimer's disease	Computer-mediated interactive voice response system with voicemail, accessed by telephone
The Alzheimer List, Washington University St. Louis MO; Funding: National Institute on Aging Alzheimer's Disease Center Grant (White & Dorman, 2000)	Alzheimer's disease	Internet mailing list (listserv) accessed by personal computer
Name, sponsorship, and funding source suppressed by researcher (Perron, 2002)	Schizophrenia and related mental health problems	Web based, accessed by personal computer

TABLE 7.1b Computer-Mediated Support Group Exemplars: Project Description and Duration/Access Information

Project Description	Duration and Access Information
ADSC: Bulletin board group, calendar, news, information on services, Q&A, chats, and links to other sites	Began as demonstration project; now on-going; Open to family caregivers; free registration required. adsc.ohioalzcenter.org
Caring-Web©: E-mail listserv group; Q&A and discussion with a nurse specialist, links to other sites	Three-month study access (concluded); restricted to research sample.
ComputerLink: Bulletin board group, e-mail, Q&A, information files, decision aid	Twelve-month study access (concluded); restricted to research sample.
Link2Care: E-mail listserv group; information files, personal journaling; Q&A; chat; links to other sites	Began as demonstration project; now ongoing; open to primary caregivers in catchment areas of California's Caregiving Resource Centers. www.link2care.net/ Link2Care/jsp/visitors_center.jsf
REACH for TLC: Telephone support group; monitoring and automated weekly caregiver's conversation with counseling, Q&A; respite conversation	18-month study (concluded); restricted to research sample.
The Alzheimer List: E-mail listserv group	Ongoing; free registration required; open to all persons with an interest in Alzheimer's disease www.adrc.wustl.edu/ALZHEIMER
Unnamed schizophrenia-focused group: Bulletin board group, e-mail	Ongoing; free registration required open to anyone with a family member with schizophrenia and related mental health problems. Address suppressed.

RESEARCH FINDINGS

FEASIBILITY

Each CMSG exemplar presented in this chapter has demonstrated the feasibility of using CMC to facilitate caregiver group support. The key references cited in Table 7.1 consistently document caregiver willingness on the part of some to use CMSGs implemented in a variety of ways and places. This is an important finding. Since the profile of the typical caregiver does not match the profile of the typical computer user, adoption of CMSGs by the intended caregiver audience must be demonstrated. Another approach to establishing feasibility involves drawing parallels between CMSG implementation and use, and theory-based features of successful technology diffusion. For example, Computer-Link caregiver participation patterns paralleled Rogers' (1983) criteria for technology diffusion (i.e., relative advantage over current methods, compatibility with lifestyle and goals, divisibility (opportunity to test component parts), low complexity and communicability (structure or effects that can be described to others) (Brennan, Moore, & Smyth, 1992). Smyth, Feinstein, and Kacerek (1997) documented that ADSC users actively modified their CMSG over time to better suit their needs, consistent with criteria identified by Rogers (1986) for adoption of communication technologies.

Moving beyond feasibility, proponents must show that CMSGs operate in a way that parallels FTF groups, and that they improve the lives of caregivers. Most studies systematically evaluating CMSG effects have focused on message content, interaction patterns, and/or impacts on caregivers' health and well-being.

MESSAGE CONTENT

Content analyses of CMSG messages have examined whether the content typifies what might be experienced in FTF support groups. Several of our exemplars have been evaluated in this way, although no two evaluations use the same set of criteria. Table 7.3 summarizes the content analysis approach taken and the key findings from each analysis. As a group, these studies support the conclusion that CMSG messages reflect interactions consistent with those found in FTF groups.

INTERACTION PATTERNS

Interaction patterns have been less frequently analyzed than message content. Smyth (1999) examined communication patterns of 13 individuals who posted 50 messages on the ADSC in a one-week period. Most could be characterized as "senders" (primarily sent messages to others) or "receivers" (primarily received messages from others). Message patterns and message content were clearly linked; users whose messages

TABLE 7.2 Computer-Mediated Support Group Message Content Analysis Approaches and Findings

Content Analyzed (Reference)	Categorization Scheme	Key Findings
ADSC: 50 bulletin board postings in one-week period (Smyth & Rose, 1998)	Theory-based support group goals, processes and benefits (Levine, 1988; Sarason & Sarason, 1985)	Both group level goals and processes and individual participant benefits identified; Psychological sense of community most frequently on the group level; Emotional expression on the individual level.
ComputerLink: 622 bulletin board postings (Brennan et al., 1995)	Themes found in FTF support groups by Toseland and Rossiter (1989)	About one third documented group/member functioning as a mutual support group system; About one quarter concerned care recipient's situation; About one fifth related to caregiving emotional impact; Others concerned developing/ using other support systems, interpersonal relationships,\ self-care, and home care skills.
Alzheimer's List: 532 list postings from first 5 days of 4 months White & Dorman, 2000)	Schema adapted from Klemm, Reppert and Visich (1998)	Over 50% of messages categorized as information giving, personal experiences, or encouragement and support.
Caring Web: group e-mailmessages (Pierce et al. 2002)	Developed from message content	Messages dealt both with general conversations about every day topics and help seeking regarding specific caregiving problems/issues.
Unnamed CMSG: 417 bulletin board postings (Perron, 2002)	10 self-help mechanisms; 16 content categories	Each self-help mechanism seen to some degree; Most common was disclosure, followed by provision of information/ advice and empathy/support; Most common content areas were emotions, diagnoses, symptoms, medications, and treatment.
Unnamed CMSG: 566 listserv messages (Mahoney, 1998)	Developed from message content; focus on issues important to family caregivers	Messages fell into three types: information seeking, information sharing, and comments; Message focus varied by stage of caregiving: Early stage—efforts to normalize the situation Middle stage—managing dementia-related problems, behavior disturbances, and medications Late stage—keeping from beingoverwhelmed by the caregiving role.

dealt with challenging caregiving issues received many more messages than they sent. Evidence of asking for and receiving within each of the individual participant support group benefits proposed by Smyth and Rose (1998) also was found. Analyzing aggregate level interaction patterns on the Alzheimer's List, White and Dorman (2000) found that within the time period under study, there were 76 information-seeking postings and 203 information-giving postings. This interaction pattern reflects the fact that multiple users frequently responded to each request for information.

Variation in Use

There is wide variation in the amount of CMSG participation among caregivers registered to use them. In their analysis of messages sent to the Alzheimer's List, White and Dorman (2000) found that a few users sent many messages, while others sent only one or two. At the time of their analysis, the list had 1,015 members, but only 178 members had posted messages. Perron (2002) found that nearly half the participants in the mental health CMSG posted only one or two messages in an 18-month observation period. Many new participants acknowledged that they had "lurked," that is, read the messages of others but not posted themselves, for some time before making their first post. Reporting on the REACH for TLC CMSG, Mahoney, Tarlow, Jones, Tennstedt, & Kasten (2001) found higher levels of use among older and better-educated caregivers, and those who reported a greater sense of management of their situation. More frequent users also were rated as highly proficient by the individuals who trained them to use the CMSG.

Impacts

Reports on the exemplars described in this chapter provide substantial anecdotal evidence of their positive impact on many caregivers. However, only two (ComputerLink and REACH for TLC) were designed to compare a group that has access to the CMSG (intervention group) with a group that does not (control group).

In the ComputerLink project, 51 caregivers randomly assigned to have access to the CMSG had improved decision-making confidence when compared with 51 caregivers who were not given access. No impact on decision-making skill or social isolation was found (Brennan, Moore, & Smyth, 1995).

Among the 51 caregivers who participated in the CMSG. Bass, McClendon, Brennan, and McCarthy (1998) found that posting to the bulletin board was associated with declines in specific types of strain for specific subgroups of caregivers. In this same sample, McClendon, Bass, Brennan, and McCarthy (1998) found that increased CMSG use led to increases in FTF support group attendance over time among caregivers who had not attended them before; among those with prior FTF group experience, CMSG use decreased FTF group attendance over time.

The REACH for TLC project was designed to investigate the impact of system use on caregiver's appraisal of the bothersome nature of caregiving, anxiety, depression, and mastery. Results showed that the intervention had a positive impact on bother from caregiving, anxiety, and depression for participants whose sense of mastery was low at the start of the project.

In a satisfaction survey, two-thirds of Link2Care users reported that it increased their knowledge about caregiving issues, and over 60% reported that it helped them to cope with caregiving and reduce feelings of isolation. Well over 80% indicated that they would recommend Link2Care to other caregivers (Kelly, Johnson, & Eskenazi, 2001).

A program evaluation survey of Alzheimer List users in 2002 found that the most appreciated features of the list were informational support (83%), sense of community (62%), and emotional support (61%). On average, users reported that use of the list had enriched their lives. Although not statistically significant, there was a trend for rural users to report the highest enrichment ratings and urban users the lowest (Meuser, personal communication).

BENEFITS AND DRAWBACKS OF CMSGS

Despite demonstrations of their feasibility and growing documentation of benefits for many of those caregivers willing to try them, CMSGs continue to remain controversial. Several CMSG benefits and drawbacks have been identified, based both on a priori assessments of CMC and actual CMSG user behavior. The positive or negative impact of some CMC features does not appear to be absolute, but dependent on the circumstances of CMSG implementation.

There is widespread agreement that certain CMSG features facilitate the receipt of social support. Chief among these are 24/7 availability, and access to the group from one's own home or another location at a personally convenient time. CMSGs can facilitate access to support by traditionally underserved populations such as the homebound, rural residents, the hearing and speech impaired, and those without reliable transportation. The pace of communication in CMSGs is generally slower than in FTF communication, and users can compose responses offline and post them whenever they wish. By promoting a more active role in self-care CMSGs also may enhance caregiver empowerment. They also may appeal to people not comfortable in FTF groups (Galinsky, Schopler, & Abell, 1997; Ripich, Moore, & Brennan, 1992; Smyth & Harris, 1993; Schopler, Abell, & Galinsky, 1998; Weinberg, Schmale, Uken, & Wessel, 1995; White & Dorman, 2000, 2001).

CMSGs also may make it easier for professionals to provide support. For example, some respondents to a survey of social workers by Galinsky, Schopler, and Abell (1997) reported that computer- and telephone-mediated groups are easier to schedule than FTF groups, and Weinberg, Schmale, Uken, and Wessel (1995) note the advantage of not having to secure a meeting place. Others have suggested that CMSGs would allow nurses to respond efficiently to multiple levels of need in multiple clients by providing emotional support, health information, and other interventions while promoting a therapeutic sense of community among them (Ripich, Moore, & Brennan, 1992; White and Dorman, 2000).

Both proponents and detractors of CMSGS share the concern that computer technology is not universally accessible. The "digital divide" keeps some caregivers from receiving support from CMSGs. Challenges include cost of equipment or Internet access, lack of computer literacy. fear of, discomfort with, or unwillingness to adapt to new technologies, limited reading or writing skills, poor vision, and poor manual dexterity (Galinsky, Schopler, & Abell, 1997; Schopler, Abell, & Galinsky, 1998; Weinberg, Schmale, Uken, & Wessel,1995; White & Dorman, 2001).

Barriers to the provision of support also have been noted. CMSGs providers are faced with the ongoing challenge of maintaining a reliable technology infrastructure and the technical support needed to deal with technology "glitches" as they arise. These challenges typically far exceed those associated with implementing FTF support groups.

CMSGs may be more difficult to moderate than FTF groups. Challenges identified include controlling negative behaviors, bringing out less "talkative" members, interpreting silence, tracking membership, and assessing member needs. Distractions in the home or in public access areas may keep caregivers from fully sharing in supportive exchanges (Galinsky, Schopler, & Abell, 1997).

A commonly cited drawback to CMSGs and most other CMC is the lack of nonverbal cues (e.g., body language, facial expression, tone of voice). This is believed to reduce "social presence," the person-oriented elements of communication such as sociability, sensitivity, warmth, and personal interest, and to make it more difficult for group members to influence one another's physiological states, feelings, and cognition (Schopler, Abell, & Galinsky, 1998; Short, Williams, & Christie, 1976; Weinberg, Schmale, Uken, & Wessel, 1995). Others argue that lack of social presence is not inherent in CMC, but dependent on the willingness of users to work at overcoming the barriers to it (Myers, 1987; Rice & Love, 1987; Walther, 1992). As Walther puts it, "as goes face-to-face goes CMC, given the opportunity for message exchange and accompanying relational development" (p. 75). Despite these assurances, some doubt that the limits of CMC can be overcome. For example, some respondents to the survey by Galinsky, Schopler, and Abell (1997) felt that CMSGs were impersonal, dehumanizing, isolating, less intimate, and less focused on interpersonal connections than FTF groups.

Some identified drawbacks of CMSGs relate to possible negative consequences of sharing personal information online, rather than to difficulties in facilitating social support per se. Confidentiality is thought to be at risk in CMSGs. As Lefton (1997) points out, however, concern for confidentiality and security of data in social services predates the Internet and the World Wide Web. These might heighten, but do not create the concern that information shared in a support group may not be held in confidence. Privacy concerns also have been raised in CMSG evaluations, i.e., CMSG users may assume that the group is more exclusive than it actually is, and reveal information that they would not typically share in a more public forum.

Providers disagree as to whether CMSGs facilitate or inhibit group process. Weinberg, Schmale, Uken, and Wessel (1995) point out that because CMSG communication is asynchronous, users lack certainty as to if or when they will receive a reply to their postings. In the survey of group workers by Galinsky, Schopler, and Abell (1997) some respondents felt that CMSG characteristics interfere with the communication process and with group bonding, delaying group cohesion and reducing provision of mutual aid and the experience of empathy. A few felt that CMSGs were antithetical to group work values. Conversely, other respondents believed that CMSGs can expedite group process by allowing members to get at issues more quickly, focus on the task, and engage in precise information exchange.

Anonymity may be the most controversial feature of CMSGs. It may facilitate social support by reducing the influence of stigma, socio-economic status, or other characteristics that might otherwise inhibit interaction. It also can allow "lurking," i.e., observing group interaction without being seen. This may let users develop a certain level of comfort before actively participating. CMSG critics fear, however, that CMSG anonymity leads to deindividuation, i.e., the submersion of oneself in the group (Kiesler, Siegel, & McGuire, 1984). Deindividuation is thought to reduce inhibitions. While this can increase idea generation and decrease conformity, it also may promote excessive levels of intimacy and impulsive, hostile, insensitive, inflammatory, or other negative behaviors. Further, "lurking" might become "social loafing," sharing in the benefits of the group without taking on the responsibilities of group membership. The impact of anonymity on receipt of social support in CMSGs may depend on the extent to which members of a CMSG participate in developing appropriate norms to govern interactions (Schopler, Abell, & Galinsky, 1998).

PRACTICE IMPLICATIONS

The growing use of CMSGs for caregivers and other target populations presents major challenges to educators and practitioners in the field. One challenge is to expand the theoretical frameworks currently guiding practice with FTF groups to accommodate CMSGs (Schopler, Abell, & Galinsky, 1998). For example, issues of physical appearance or attraction, physical proximity, and frequent interaction dominate theories of relational development. However, the construction of most of these theories predates the advent of CMC. (Parks and Floyd, 1996).

A second challenge is teaching service providers to exploit the benefits and circumvent the drawbacks of CMSGs. They must learn how to select, use, and become comfortable with CMSG technology. This requires the creation of practice guidelines at several levels: 1) pre-implementation (e.g., integrating CMSGs within the larger agency or organization, securing adequate technology and technical support; choosing appropriate target groups; specifying group composition and size; determining amount and type of monitoring needed); 2) implementation (e.g., assessing individuals for membership and preparing them for participation; establishing group norms regarding privacy, lurking, etc.); 3) managing group process (e.g., compensating for lack of nonverbal cues; coaching users on preserving desired anonymity while fostering cohesion; establishing procedures for welcoming and integrating new members; and drawing "lurkers" into the group) (Galinsky, Schopler, & Abell, 1997; Schopler, Abell, & Galinsky, 1988; White and Dorman, 2001).

CONCLUSIONS

Much has been learned since the emergence of CMC and its initial CMSG applications. Feasibility has been documented. Thousands have used CMSGs and provided anecdotal evidence of their benefits. Yet, little is known about the caregiver characteristic associated with CMSGs use or why volume of use varies so widely among group members (White & Dorman, 2001). Additional studies of these issues will help in targeting and customizing CMSG use, and they also will help to identify and overcome barriers to use. While anticipated advances in CMC and closing of the "digital divide" will remove some barriers to use in the future, studies are urgently needed because the needs of the elderly and their caregivers must be better served now.

To inform practice guidelines, studies of both process and outcome are needed. In particular randomized trials are needed to establish CMSG efficacy and their effectiveness under "real world" conditions. If potential subjects are first screened for their willingness to use CMSGs before being randomly assigned to experimental and control conditions, these studies also might help to disentangle issues of readiness to use technology from other influences on the amount of use caregivers make of a CMSG and the impacts of CMSG use on caregiver well-being. Hard empirical evidence of effectiveness is also needed if CMC technology is to be routinely underwritten by local, state, or national governments, health care providers, and the like in support of organizational and individual health care and social services goals.

CMSG studies suffer from a lack of agreed upon criteria to demonstrate that CMSGs are adequate substitutes for FTF support groups. As noted above, several options are already available in the literature. Measures that establish what elements of social support are important to CMSG users are also needed (see Smyth & Rose, 2002). One of the fears associated with CMC is that it will be used as a complete substitution for FTF contacts. We believe that this is a serious issue to be dealt with now, but that it will recede as the quality of social interaction via CMC begins to approximate communication by nontechnological means.

Most formally evaluated CMSGs have been time limited, grant supported endeavors. Providers of ongoing CMSGs (e.g., the ADSC, the Alzheimer List and Link2Care) have had to work diligently to maintain funding to support these efforts. While technological advances have paved the way for creative enhancements of CMSGs, they also have increased the need for technical expertise and more sophisticated end-user equipment. CMSGs are thought to cost less than FTF groups and to increase client empowerment by reducing their reliance on health care (Galinsky, Schopler, & Abell, 1997), but there have been no cost-effectiveness studies to date. In the future, we can expect wider availability of devices that are more portable, more affordable, and easier to use then current personal computer technology. These developments will no doubt improve our ability to enhance technology-based information and support interventions.

In short, the use of CMSGs for family caregivers holds great promise. Realizing that promise will require diligence on the part of practitioners and researchers alike. We also believe that CMC use should not be limited to compensating for unmet needs of older persons, but should be exploited for the contribution it can make to universal access to resources and enhanced social participation.

ACKNOWLEDGMENTS

Kathleen A. Smyth is Associate Professor and Acting Director, Division of Health Services Research, Department of Epidemiology and Biostatistics, Case Western Reserve University School of Medicine, Cleveland, Ohio. Sunkyo Kwon is affiliated with the Graduate School of Applied Gerontology, Sookmyung University, Seoul, Republic of Korea (South).

REFERENCES

Alzheimer's Association (1995). *Support group manual.* Chicago: Author.

Bass, D. M., McClendon, M. J., Brennan, P. F., & McCarthy, C. (1998). The buffering effect of a computer support network on caregiver strain. *Journal of Aging and Health, 10*(2), 20–43.

Berge, Z. L. (1994). Electronic discussion groups. *Communication Education, 43,* 102–111.

Bourgeois, M. S., & Schulz, R. (1996). Interventions for caregivers of patients with Alzheimer's disease: A review and analysis of content, process, and outcomes. *International Journal of Aging and Human Development, 43*(1), 35–92.

Brennan, P. F., Moore, S. M., & Smyth, K. A. (1992). Alzheimer's disease caregivers' uses of a computer network. *Western Journal of Nursing Research, 14*(5), 662–663.

Brennan, P. F., Moore, S. M., & Smyth, K. A. (1995). The effects of a special computer network on caregivers of persons with Alzheimer's disease. *Nursing Research, 44*(3), 166–172.

Caregivers of those with Alzheimer's (1999). *Report of findings.* Bethesda: National Alliance for Caregiving.

National Academy on an Aging Society (2000). Caregiving: Helping the elderly with activity limitations. Report #7. Washington, DC: Author. Available at: www.agingsociety.org/agingsociety/pdf/Caregiving.pdf

Frankel, M. S., & Siang, S. (1999). *Ethical and legal aspects of human subjects research on the Internet.* New York: American Association for the Advancement of Science. Available at: www.aaas.org/spp/dspp/sfrl/projects/intres/main.htm

Galinsky, M. J., Schopler, J. H., & Abell, M. D. (1997). Connecting group members through telephone and computer groups. *Health & Social Work, 22*(3), 181–188.

Gonyea, J. G. (1989). Alzheimer's disease support groups: An analysis of their structure, format and perceived benefits. *Social Work in Health Care, 14*(1), 61–72.

Henderson, J. N., Gutierrez-Mayka, M., Garcia, J., & Boyd, S. (1993). A model for Alzheimer's disease support group development in African-American and Hispanic populations. *Gerontologist, 33*(3), 409–414.

Kelly, K., Johnson, P., & Eskenazi, L. (2001, March). Lessons from the field: Implementation of Link2Care, an Internet-based services program. Presented at the Joint Conference of the American Society on Aging and the National Council on the Aging, New Orleans.

Kiesler, S., Siegel, J., & McGuire, T. W. (1984). Social psychological aspects of computer-mediated communication. *American Psychologist, 39,* 1123–1134.

King, S. A., & Moreggi, D. (1998). Internet therapy and self-help groups: The pros and cons. In J. Gackenbach (Ed.), *Psychology and the Internet.* New York: Academic Press.

Lefton, A. B. (1997). Confidentiality and security in information technology. *Generations,* Fall, 50–52.

Mahoney, D. F. (1998). A content analysis of an Alzheimer family caregivers virtual focus group. *American Journal of Alzheimer's Disease, 13*(6), 309–316.

Mahoney, D. M. F., Tarlow, B., Jones, R. N., Tennstedt, S., & Kasten, L. (2001). Factors affecting the use of a telephone-based intervention for caregivers of people with Alzheimer's disease. *Journal of Telemedicine and Telecare, 7*(3), 139–148.

McClendon, M. J., Bass, D. M., Brennan, P. F., & McCarthy, C. (1998). A computer network for Alzheimer's caregivers and use of support group services. *Journal of Aging and Health, 4 (Winter),* 403–420.

McConnell, S., & Riggs, J. A. (1994). A public policy agenda supporting family caregiving. In M. H. Cantor (Ed.), *Family caregiving agenda for the future*. San Francisco: American Society on Aging.

McKenna, K. Y. A., & Bargh, J. A. (1998). Coming out in the age of the Internet: Identity 'de-marginalization' from virtual group participation. *Journal of Personality and Social Psychology, 75*(3), 681–694.

Myers, D. (1987). "Anonymity is part of the magic": Individual manipulation of computer-mediated communication contexts. *Qualitative Sociology, 10*(3), 251–266.

Parks, M. R., & Floyd, K. (1996). Making friends in cyberspace. *Journal of Communication, 46*(1), 80–97.

Perron, B. (2002). Online support for caregivers of people with a mental illness. *Psychiatric Rehabilitation Journal, 26*(1), 70–77.

A portrait of informal caregivers in America. (2001). Portland: The Foundation for Accountability and the Robert Wood Johnson Foundation.

Pross, H. (1972). *Medienforschung [Media Research]*. Darmstadt, Germany: Wissenschaftliche Buchgesellschaft.

Rice, R. E., & Love, G. (1987). Electronic emotion: Socioemotional content in a computer-mediated communication network. *Communications Research, 14*(1), 85–108.

Ripich, S., Moore, S. M., & Brennan, P. F. (1992). A new nursing medium: Computer networks for group interaction. *Journal of Psychosocial Nursing and Mental Health Services, 30*, 15–20.

Rogers, E. (1983). *Diffusion of innovations* (3rd ed.). New York: The Free Press.

Rogers, E. M. (1986). *Communication technology: The new media in society.* New York: The Free Press.

Schmall, V. L. (1984). It doesn't just happen: What makes a support group good? *Generations, 9*, 64–67.

Schopler, J. H., Abell, M. D., & Galinsky, M. J. (1998). Technology-based groups: A review and conceptual framework for practice. *Social Work, 43*(3), 254–267.

Schulz, R., O'Brien, B. S., Bookwala, J., & Fleissner, K. (1995). Psychiatric and physical morbidity effects of dementia caregiving: Prevalence, correlates, and causes. *Gerontologist, 35*, 771–791.

Short, J., Williams, W., & Christie, B. (1976). *The Social Psychology of Telecommunications*. London: Wiley.

Smyth, K. A. (1999). Computer-assisted qualitative analysis of computer-mediated communication. Program Abstracts. *Gerontologist, 39* (Special Issue 1), 64.

Smyth, K. A., Feinstein, S. J., & Kacerek, S. (1997). The Alzheimer's disease support center: Information and support for family caregivers through computer mediated communication. In P. Brennan, S. J. Schneider, & E. Tornquist (Eds.), *Community health care information networks*. New York: Springer Publishing.

Smyth, K. A., & Harris, P. B. (1993). Using telecomputing to provide information and support to caregivers of persons with dementia. *Gerontologist, 33*(1), 123–127.

Smyth, K. A., & Rose, J. H. (1998). Can caregiver support group goals, processes and benefits be achieved through computer-mediated communication? Program Abstracts. *Gerontologist, 38* (Special Issue 1), 345.

Smyth, K. A., & Rose, J. H. (2002). Measuring impacts of computer-mediated support for family caregivers. Program Abstracts. *Gerontologist, 42* (Special Issue 1), 286.

Vrooman, S. S. (2002). The art of invective: Performing identity in cyberspace. *New Media and Society, 4*(1), 41–70.

Walther, J. B. (1992). Interpersonal effects in computer-mediated interaction: A relational perspective. *Communication Research, 19*(1), 52–90.

Weinberg, N., Schmale, J. D., Uken, J., & Wessel, K. (1995). Computer-mediated support groups. *Social Work with Groups, 17*(4), 43–54.

White, M. H., & Dorman, S. M. (2000). Online support for caregivers: Analysis of an Internet Alzheimer mail group. *Computers in Nursing, 18,* 168–176.

White, M., & Dorman, S. M. (2001). Receiving social support online: Implications for health education. *Health Education Research Theory and Practice, 16*(6), 693–707.

The wide circle of caregiving: Key findings from a national survey: Long-term care from the caregiver's perspective. (2002). Menlo Park: The Henry J. Kaiser Family Foundation.

Wright, S. D., Lund, D. A., Pett, M. A., & Caserta, M. S. (1987). The assessment of support group experience by caregivers of dementia patients. *Clinical Gerontologist, 6,* 35–59.

Section C

Assistive Technology in the
Home and Environment

8

Assistive Technology as Tools for Everyday Living and Community Participation While Aging

Joy Hammel

To start this introductory chapter on assistive technology (AT), I will use a personal example to illustrate the power of AT and issues related to its use. My parents are currently in their late 70s and early 80s. During the past 10 years, they've experienced several aging and disability-related issues. As an occupational therapist specializing in AT, I have brought many types of AT for them to try. For most, they have politely declined, telling me that I could give them to "some other disabled person who could use it." Some AT, however, was an instant hit, such as a foldable cane, a pill splitter/crusher, a portable amplifier unit, and a tub bench. After dad's back surgery, the occupational therapist left him with a number of AT devices, but with no instructions for their use. Dad left all but the reacher at the hospital and said "Mom will help me." Recently, they've struggled with the decision whether to stay in their home of 50 years, or to move. I offered to help them adapt their home and strategize supports to manage. They politely declined and chose to move to a senior independent living community, noting that they'd rather live someplace where they had control as opposed to someplace where they would need help from others. They found a nice apartment in a large complex with many supports; however, I was chagrined to note many environmental shortcomings. The contractors installed prefabricated fiberglass shower/tub inserts, leaving a 3-inch difference in height between the tub and the floor, a safety issue even for me. The grab bar mounted outside the unit was too far away to be useful. The washcloth holder looked like a grab bar, and was being used as one by my parents, but would not support anyone's full weight. I had other concerns with lighting, room temperature, storage location, and flooring. Still, overall, my parents seem happy with the living situation because it's manageable and they can get out and roam around the community. Of note, every time I go over, I see more AT, often products that other neighbors have introduced them to that they like and pick up from local stores. They then pass these ideas onto to other people in the building—a kind of strategy-trading network. They occasionally ask me for advice, but like to look at catalogues and think about ideas I leave with them and then make a decision.

This example from my life demonstrates many of the pros, cons, and issues to consider with assistive technology (AT), particularly when focusing on it through the lens of aging. My parents, and their interaction with AT and with me, are perfect illustrations of issues related to:

- the close interaction of AT, and the decision to use it or not, with the physical environment and social world surrounding people
- physical assistance as opposed to, or in conjunction with, AT
- needing or asking for help and what that means to older adults in our society, which places a high value on independence as "doing completely by yourself"
- resistance to being stigmatized as "handicapped" or disabled
- safety and security without compromising choice, control, and dignity
- professionals or family determining AT needs versus consumer choice or learning about AT via social learning with peers
- changing needs, and whether environments and technologies accommodate those needs
- interdependence and social needs, preferences, and desires to participate in the community beyond basic activities of daily living
- society continuing to plan and build spaces and technologies that do not promote continued participation, or meet the preferences and needs of the aging and aged

This section of this book (as well as the chapters by Dienel, Peine, and Cameron, and by Watzke in the following section) focuses on many of these issues and complexities of AT. It presents many innovative examples of AT-related products, environmental adaptations, and methods for designing and researching AT use, many of which describe promising strategies and trends, all of which raise even more issues and challenges from the aging community for those of us in the AT or gerotechnology field. This chapter places AT in context, summarizes what we know and are learning about AT use, particularly in regard to aging, and presents ideas for future directions and research, development, and service delivery.

TRENDS IN ASSISTIVE TECHNOLOGY, TECHNOLOGY, AND THE ENVIRONMENT

To frame the discussion, we first need to think: What is AT? When you hear the words "assistive technology," many people think of wheelchairs, walkers, and canes. However, this definition was expanded broadly by legislation to include "any item, piece of equipment or product systems, whether acquired commercially off the shelf, modified, or customized, that is used to increase, maintain, or improve functional capabilities of individuals with disabilities" (Public Law 105–394, 1998). Interestingly, when older adults with disabilities were asked what assistive devices are most important to them they identify very basic categories across a range of uses (Mann, Llanes, Justiss, & Tomita, 2003). The top five most important devices cited were eyeglasses, canes, wheelchairs, walkers, and phones. When controlled for the number of people using the device, the top five were oxygen tanks, dentures, 3-in-1 commodes, computers, and wheelchairs.

Typically we group AT into categories related to seating/positioning/mobility, access (environmental control, computer), communication, and sensory technologies. Changes or modifications in the physical *and* social environment occur with the introduction of any technology, and introduce new functional categories including home modifications (e.g., grab bars, ramps, lifts, and accessible entryways), and worksite accommodations (such as ergonomically designed computer interfaces and workstations).

Several trends have caused us to broaden AT beyond the traditional categories. Two related environmental design approaches, universal design (Connell, Jones, Mace, Mueller, Mullick, et al., 1997) and design of age-friendly/elder-ready communities (Elderberry Institute, 2003), have challenged the notion of "assistive" as a separate category. They both seek to broaden design of technologies and environments to be "usable by all people, to the greatest extent possible, without the need for adaptation or specialized design" (Mace, Hardie, & Place, 1996). In response, a host of "universally designed products" are appearing on the market, such as easy grip cooking utensils. We are now seeing the design of entire communities that have built-in features that allow people to "age in place," including transportation, communication, and social participation opportunities designed to meet the expressed needs of seniors and, in some cases, to promote intergenerational social learning and support to seniors so they feel like a part of the community (Elderberry Institute, 2003).

The explosion of information technology (e.g., computers, Internet, personal digital assistants, and integrated phone/communication/computer systems) has also created a new and rapidly growing area of technology development. The older adult population increasingly goes "online" to seek out health information, purchase products, pursue interests, and engage in social networking. This is reflected in the success of SeniorNet (www.seniornet.org/php/), a national network of computer/Internet training centers. Legislation including the Telecommunications Act (Section 255) and the Rehabilitation Act (Section 508) now expand this access, mandating that these technologies be accessible to aging and disabled consumers. IBM has linked with SeniorNet and the American Society on Aging to offer Web adaptations for seniors, such as enlarged text, reduced clutter, and mouse adaptations (www.seniornet.org/ibm/).

In concert with information and networking technology advancement, there is also a trend in areas such as telemedicine, telerehabilitation, and telehealth, where consumers can interact with and solve problems in consultation with health care providers without having to leave their homes. Blending telerehabilitation, information technology, and assistive technology, we see increasingly sophisticated examples of "Smart Houses," Personal Emergency Response Systems (PERS), and Automated Activity Track and Analysis Systems (AATAS), as described by Kutzik and Glascock and by Parker and Sabata in this section.

All of these technologies and trends may merge when we discuss "assistive technology" as a broad concept; when applied to older adults the terms "gerotechnology" or "gerontechnology" have also been used.

For the purposes of this chapter, the term "assistive technology and environmental interventions" (AT-EI) will be used to describe the range of products, devices, equipment, technologies, and the environmental features, modifications, and designs that may be used by older adults and those aging with disabilities to meet several daily living, health and wellness, communication, mobility, control, and social participation needs.

ASSISTIVE TECHNOLOGY: THE POSITIVE IMPACT

Several studies have shown the benefits of AT use by older adults and people aging with disabilities. Mann, Ottenbacher, Fraas, Tomita, and Granger, (1999) examined the effect of AT-EI with 100 frail elders in a randomized controlled trial, comparing persons who received functional and home assessments with AT-EI to address issues, with those who received usual home care services. Although both groups showed functional declines within 18 months, there were significantly more declines in the control group, and hospital and nursing home costs were more than three times higher for the control group.

In another randomized controlled trial (Gitlin, Corcoran, Winter, Boyce, & Hauck, 2001), older adults with Alzheimer's disease and their spouse caregivers receiving a client-centered environmental intervention in the home were compared with those receiving usual care services. Intervention was based upon Lawton's Person/Environment Competence Model (1982), and used an approach in which occupational therapists worked with older adults and caregivers to plan and implement physical and social environmental strategies to accommodate changing functional needs. Treatment group caregivers reported fewer declines in clients' IADLs, fewer declines in self-care, and fewer behavior problems at 3 months post treatment (Gitlin, Corcoran, Winter, Boyce & Hauck, 2001). Caregivers in the treatment group reported less upset, women caregivers reported increased self-efficacy in managing behaviors, and women and minority caregivers reported improved self-efficacy in managing functional issues. This research has led to the validation of new instruments for evaluating person-environment fit (Gitlin, Schinfeld, Winter, Corcoran, Boyce, et al., 2002), and begins to illuminate a positive "spread effect" in that environmental strategies support not only individual users but also others in their social world, such as family and caregivers.

Hammel, Lai, and Heller (2002) evaluated the additive impact of later life AT-EI on function and community living in a longitudinal study of 109 people with developmental disabilities who were who were trying to transition to community settings from institutional ones and experiencing age and disability-related issues. Results indicated a supportive buffer effect of AT in maintaining or improving function over time for people living in the community and nursing homes, although people in the community had more support to engage in a wider range of activities beyond basic ADLs. In a follow-up intervention study, Hammel and Nochajski applied Gitlin's environmental intervention approach to people aging with developmental disabilities and important others, including family, staff, peers, and caregivers (Heller, Janicki, Hammel, & Factor, 2002). The program was expanded to include disability activists working with consumers to strategize system and societal level barriers to AT use, such as funding, attitudes, and protocols/regulations of the group home environment. Preliminary findings indicate a similar spread effect when introducing environmental strategies within a group setting. Peers and staff saw the positive effects of the AT-EI as the consumer used it, began to validate the person and view them as a mentor/role model, and then began to use the same strategy or ask to replicate it themselves. For example, environmental modifications to a shared bathroom space to improve access and function for one consumer were used by all other residents of that group home, and also supported staff in reducing the level of assistance, and giving more control to residents in the everyday routines.

In chapters throughout this book many other examples demonstrate the positive impact of AT-EI. Parker and Sabata, and Kutzik and Glascock provide numerous examples of supportive AT for home access, automation, monitoring, and safety/security. They also discuss examples of integrated AT systems that interface with computers, e-mail, the Web, and other remote networking technology to serve multiple purposes, including emergency communication with family or emergency response services, and ongoing tracking of changing health, medical, or functional needs through telehealth/rehabilitative technologies that help flag or prevent accidents (e.g., falls, over- or undermedication, wandering) or functional declines that may otherwise result in nursing home placements. These technologies can help older adults stay in their homes, and also support family, personal attendant/in-home supports, and health care professionals. Parker and Sabata also discuss the community-integrated residential environments designed to be more like home and to support individual choice and control within an assisted living setting.

Watzke provides several examples of AT development within the Living Laboratory that also use Lawton's (1982) model. These include improved interfaces to personal digital assistants (PDAs) and environmental daily living devices (EDLDs), and research on the effectiveness of devices to prevent injury among workers/caregivers, including more effective and efficient lifting and transferring devices. Watzke also discusses the "crossover potential" in utilizing technology developed with the younger disability community or within other industries, and applying them to the aging market. He cites examples of using EDL technology used by people with high-level spinal cord injuries as being applied and customized for older adults to monitor their homes and security within them. There are many other examples of security, defense, and telecommunications technologies that have only begun to be explored with seniors.

ISSUES WITH AT AND AGING

Given the growing research on AT-EI that supports its positive effects, several questions emerge: Why aren't more seniors and people aging with disabilities using AT-EI? What causes people to not use, or to abandon or reject AT-EI? and Why aren't more environments and technologies being designed to reflect the needs of seniors and people aging with disabilities? These questions bring us to the heart of several issues regarding AT access and use.

AT ABANDONMENT

Significant rates of AT abandonment have been shown in general, and specifically among older adults (Gitlin, Schemm, Landsberg, & Burgh, 1996; Philips & Zhao, 1993). Gitlin's (1995) summary of why older adults reject technology points to reasons at several levels, including the person (perceived need, functional status, and perceptions of disability related to use of devices), environmental (physical and social factors influencing device use), the device (aesthetics, quality, durability, ease of use, fit to person and context), and the sociocultural context. A central factor in abandonment is lack of consumer involvement and control in the AT decision-making process. The need to involve older adults as informed consumers in the AT design and delivery process is critical. Dienel and Cameron propose a participatory approach to designing and assessing AT needs in which older adults are actively involved in all stages of decision making from needs assessment through product evaluation.

THE INTERPLAY OF NEED & ECONOMICS

Although abandonment research provides insights into why older adults are not using AT, evidence suggests they are not obtaining needed AT-EI in the first place. This unmet need is growing as the older adult population expands and younger people with disabilities begin to age. Less than 10% of all persons age 65–74, and less than 15% of those 75 and older have home modifications (LaPlante, Hendershot, and Moss, 1997). Less than one-third of seniors with disabilities have adapted the most common home issues (e.g., grab bars, ramps, wide doors, and raised toilets) (Mutschler and Miller, 1991). Less than 37% of older adults reporting limitations in bathing and toileting reported use of adaptive equipment such as tub seats, grab bars, and raised toilet seats (Manton, Corder & Stallard, 1993). Although the number of seniors using computer technologies is increasing in general, only 10.6% of seniors with disabilities have computers, and only 2.2% report Internet access (Kaye, 2000).

Studies of AT-EI access and use suggest that cost and lack of sufficient financial resources or supports to pay for needed technology are key factors. An estimated 2.5 million Americans report needing AT but being unable to obtain it, mostly due to affordability (LaPlante, Hendershot, and Moss, 1997). In a study examining whether AT could substitute for personal assistance services, researchers found that Medicaid recipients or those who were poor were more likely to use no AT or only some AT for specific ADLs (Hoenig, Taylor, & Sloan, 2003). This finding further suggests that economic status, often correlated with disability status and race, impacts basic access to AT and suppresses potential benefits that could be gained from its use.

These findings clearly indicate the need to emphasize systems change in funding AT-and effective systems and programs for delivering AT to older adults with limited financial resources. For example, the AT Alternative Financing Program (AFP) currently offered in 14 states offers reduced interest rates, flexible terms, and guaranteed loan programs to people with disabilities of any age within a consumer-directed approach similar to applying for a bank loan (see www.resna.org/). A few states such as Maryland and Georgia have targeted AT delivery to low-income seniors with high AT need through Area Agencies on Aging; there is much room for growth in information, training, demonstration centers, and community-based delivery of AT to low-income older adults (Cavanaugh & Emerman, 1996).

USE ISSUES: AT VERSUS PERSONAL ASSISTANCE

Intimately related to cost and to AT use are issues surrounding the complex web of help, physical assistance, and independence/dependence in our society. In their analysis of the 1994 National Long Term Care Survey, Hoenig, Taylor, and Sloan (2003) found the use of equipment associated with fewer hours of help. Verbrugge and Sevak (2002) examined AT and personal assistance strategies among older adults with disabilities, finding equipment was more effective than personal assistance in improving independence (defined as ability to perform ADLs), reporting that equipment may offer the added benefits of customization, availability, and increased self sufficiency to the user

Yet, other research by Kincade Norburn and colleagues (1995) demonstrated that people who received assistance from others were more likely to engage in self-care activities themselves; thus, assistance can be interpreted as a social support rather than a problem or a burden. The issue of AT replacing personal assistance is complex. A number of questions arise:

- Can AT-EI by itself replace human supports for a length of time, under what conditions or for what activities, and at what cost to the person in relation to time and energy?
- What are the person's preferences in relation to use of AT and/or personal assistance? Are there certain tasks or time blocks during which they'd prefer to have one or the other, or a combination of the two? Do they have preferences about when they would like to be self sufficient versus when they would prefer help?
- What happens when an older adult needs physical assistance in addition to AT? If we begin a dynamic of looking at hours or cost savings, will a person with higher functional needs be able to get both, or will funding only be allocated for one or the other and the older adult forced to choose, or not be given a choice, if there are cost differences?

We know very little about these issues, particularly older adults' preferences, in our current research. The disability community has raised these issues often, as they question whether AT and personal assistance should be an either/or situation, or one of personal choice.

Another issue is the complexity of physical help when viewed in the context of social interaction, relationships, and interdependence. Most research on AT with older adults has been specific to AT as an assist with basic ADLs (e.g., toileting, transferring), with an emphasis on the goal of performing by oneself without help. For the many older adults and people aging with disabilities, independence as defined in this way is not the goal, nor is that goal achievable with only AT-EI in many cases. Instead, independence, as defined by freedom and choice in deciding what, how, when, and with whom, becomes central. This reconceptualization of independence focuses on a much broader range of AT-EI as well, including technology and environmental modifications to support community living over institutionalization, and to support social participation, interaction, inclusion, and communication above and beyond basic ADLs. We have just begun exploring the application and impact of technologies such as computers and Internet as health tools with the aging and disabled. We have yet to examine whether access to technologies such as computers/Internet and adapted transportation may also lead to increased social participation that in turn helps people remain more active and invested in the world around them, resulting in many unrealized benefits above and beyond physical independence.

SAFETY & SECURITY: AT WHAT COST TO PRIVACY, CHOICE, AND DIGNITY?

Another related issue is that of AT as a safety tool. Many of the technologies described throughout this book are intended to help people remain in their homes by addressing safety and security issues. The environmental strategies used by Gitlin and colleagues with older adults with Alzheimer's disease helped to relieve caregiver upset by providing more options to respond to behavioral issues via the environment or technologies in it. The EDLs and home automation described by several authors in this book help to control the environment, freeing people from that responsibility and helping them to feel more secure. However, as we begin to apply more technology to regulate and monitor the environment and people's actions within it, we also begin to encounter issues of privacy, control, choice, and dignity. Questions concerning whether people want their entire house wired and monitored, what activities are monitored and how, where the information gathered goes and who sees it or has access to it, whether the consumer has the choice to turn it off when privacy is desired, and what happens to it in relation to decisions about whether a person can stay in the home or not and related decisions (e.g., continued insurance coverage), begin to arise as well. This is an area for future study, particularly using participatory methods of the type described by Dienel and Cameron in the next section that actively involve older adults in the design.

CONCLUSIONS

Clearly, assistive technology and related environmental strategies are valuable tools for supporting, and perhaps enabling, community living and participation with older adults and people aging with disabilities. AT-EI has been found to benefit functional maintenance and improvement, self efficacy, and social participation for older adults, as well as provide benefits to family, caregivers, peers, and service providers who interact closely with older adults in their everyday lives. New applications of gerotechnology, such as automated activity tracking and analysis systems, and integrated telecommunications/home automation systems offer strategies for older adults to stay in their homes and to age in place. However, key issues related to unmet needs, economic barriers to access, AT abandonment, AT versus personal assistance, and safety at a cost to privacy and control need to be seriously considered at the same time that new technology is developed. Methods of participatory research enable older adults to actively participate in technology and environmental design, creation, and evaluation within future research and development efforts, offering a valuable methodology. Additionally, systems change initiatives to build more accessible technologies and create universally designed communities that enable people to age in place yet still remain a vital part of the community, and systems and programs that inform older adults and people aging with disability about AT-EI options and link them to funding and consumer-directed delivery systems all offer promising areas for future growth and development.

ACKNOWLEDGMENTS

Joy Hammel is Assistant Professor in the Department of Occupational Therapy/Disability and Human Development, University of Illinois at Chicago.

REFERENCES

Cavanaugh, G., & Emerman, J. (1996). *Assistive technology and home modification project report.* San Francisco, CA: American Society on Aging.

Connell, B. R., Jones, M., Mace, R., Mueller, J., Mullick, A., Ostroff, E., et al. (1997). *The principles of universal design.* Raleigh, NC: North Carolina State University Center for Universal Design.

Elderberry Institute (2003). *Is my community elder-friendly?* St. Paul, MN: Author.

Gitlin, L. N. (1995). Why older people accept or reject assistive technology. *Generations, 19(1),* 41–46.

Gitlin, L. N., Corcoran, M., Winter, L., Boyce, A., & Hauck, W. W. (2001). Randomized, controlled trial of a home environmental intervention: Effect on efficacy and upset in caregivers and on daily function of persons with dementia. *Gerontologist, 41(1),* 4–14.

Gitlin, L. N., Schemm, R. L., Landsberg, L., & Burgh, D. (1996). Factors predicting assistive device use in the home by older people following rehabilitation. *Journal of Aging and Health, 8(4),* 554–575.

Gitlin, L. N., Schinfeld, S., Winter, L., Corcoran, M., Boyce, A. A., & Hauck, W. (2002). Evaluating home environments of persons with dementia: Interrater reliability and validity of the Home Environmental Assessment Protocol (HEAP). *Disability and Rehabilitation, 24(1–3),* 59–71.

Hammel, J., Lai, J., & Heller, T. (2002). The impact of assistive technology and environmental interventions on function and living situation status for people who are aging with developmental disabilities. *Disability and Rehabilitation, 24(1–3),* 93–105.

Heller, T., Janicki, M., Hammel, J., & Factor, A. (2002). *Promoting healthy aging, family support, and age-friendly communities for persons aging with developmental disabilities: Report of the 2001 Invitational Research Symposium on Aging with Developmental Disabilities.* Chicago, IL: University of Illinois-Chicago Rehabilitation Research ant Technology Center on Aging and Developmental Disability.

Hoenig, H., Taylor, D., & Sloan, F. (2003). Does assistive technology substitute for personal assistance among the disabled elderly? *American Journal of Public Health, 93(2),* 330–337.

Kaye, H. S. (2000). *Computer and Internet use among people with disabilities: Disability statistics report (13).* Washington DC: U.S. Department of Education, National Institute on Disability and Rehabilitation Research.

Kincade Norburn, J. E., Bernard, S. L., Konrad, T. R., Woomert, A., DeFriese, G. H., Kalsbeek, et al. (1995). Self-care and assistance from others in coping with functional status limitations among a national sample of older adults. *Journal of Gerontology, 50B(2),* 101–109.

LaPlante, M. P., Hendershot, G. E., & Moss, A. J. (1997). The prevalence of need for assistive technology devices and home accessibility features. *Technology & Disability, 6(1/2),* 17–28.

Lawton, M. P. (1982). Competence, environmental press and the adaptation of older people. In M. P. Lawton, P. G. Windley, & T. O. Byerts (Eds.), *Aging and the environment.* New York: Springer Publishing.

Mace, R., Hardie, G., & Place, J. (1996). *Accessible environments: Toward universal design.* Raleigh, NC: Center for Universal Design, North Carolina State University.

Mann, W. C., Llanes, C., Justiss, M. D., & Tomita, M. (2003). Frail elders' self report of their most important assistive devices. Gainesville, FL: Rehabilitation Engineering Research Center on Aging.

Mann, W. C., Ottenbacher, K. J., Fraas, L., Tomita, M., & Granger, C. V. (1999). Effectiveness of assistive technology and environmental interventions in maintaining independence and reducing home care costs for the frail elderly: A randomized controlled trial. *Archives of Family Medicine, 8,* 210–217.

Manton, K. G., Corder, L., & Stallard, E. (1993). Changes in the use of personal assistance and special equipment from 1982 to 1989: Results from the 1982 and 1989 National Long Term Care Survey. *Gerontologist, 33*(2), 168–174.

Mutschler, P. H., & Miller, J. R. (1991, November). *Staying put: Adapting to frailty in owner occupied housing.* Paper presented at the Annual Meeting of the Gerontological Society of America, Minneapolis, Minnesota.

Philips, B., & Zhao, H. (1993). Predictors of assistive technology abandonment. *Assistive Technology, 5,* 36–45.

Public Law 105–394 (1998). *The Assistive Technology Act of 1998.* Washington DC: Congressional Report.

Verbrugge, L., & Sevak, P. (2002). Use, type, and efficacy of assistance for disability. *Journal of Gerontology Social Sciences, 57B*(6), S366–S379.

9

Monitoring Household Occupant Behaviors to Enhance Safety and Well-Being

*David M. Kutzik and
Anthony P. Glascock*

THE RATIONALE FOR AUTOMATED
ACTIVITY TRACKING AND ANALYSIS SYSTEMS

Automated Activity Tracking and Analysis Systems (AATAS) provide a technological solution to one of the most vexing problems facing caregivers and case managers: not having objective, timely information on the activities and functional status of at-risk older persons, especially those living alone. Knowing if an older person is up and around in her/his home, preparing meals, managing medications and, moreover, maintaining a normal level of activities is essential for effective caregiving. Until recently, caregivers and providers have had to rely on short visits, direct observations, and repeated questioning of the older person about her/his activities to gain insight into her/his daily activities and to identify possible areas of difficulty. Even when undertaken, there are severe limitations in each of these approaches, but they can be overcome by the use of an AATAS.

In principal, any routine daily activity can be monitored as long as it entails patterned interaction with objects in the home environment. Through the use of Internet-based telecommunications, AATAS allow for

132

repeated "checking in" on the monitored individual from any remote location. Using software capable of identifying subtle changes in the frequency, timing, and duration of specific activities, it is possible for AATAS to detect changes in behavior that may signal changes in functional and medical status before they become a crisis (Glascock & Kutzik, 2000).

AATAS TECHNOLOGY AND FUNCTIONING

The core concept of Automated Activity Tracking and Analysis is behavioral monitoring, especially the tracking of core functional activities, i.e., ADLs and IADLs. It is therefore useful to describe in some detail the configuration of a monitoring system. AATAS comprises three subsystems: 1) an in-home monitor consisting of a data acquisition unit and an array of sensors in the home of the monitored individual; 2) a Web site that provides for processing of the sensor data converting them to behavioral information which is displayed with graphics and text; and, 3) the remote caregiver's terminal or interface.

IN-HOME DATA COLLECTOR

The in-home data collector subsystem, consisting of an array of sensors and a base station, can be seen in the right side of Figure 9.1. Small wireless sensors are placed throughout the home to detect motion, the opening and closing of doors and drawers, as well as more specialized actions, such as the removal and replacement of medications from containers. Signals from these sensors are received by the base station unit, which stores and periodically uploads the data to the remote monitoring site on the Internet. The home base station unit comprises a wireless data receiver, a computer used for data storage, low-level processing and Internet upload, and a modem.

Installations vary with the layout of the individual house or apartment, but typically consist of motion detectors both in and between the bathroom and bedroom, a door opening sensor on the refrigerator and/or microwave, a flush detector in the toilet, and a medication pill or bottle holder which detects medication usage by means of sensors capable of signaling removal and replacement of the medication. Since the small wireless sensor devices can literally be put in place with Velcro or double-sided tape, it is possible to avoid expensive and disruptive retrofitting, and reduce installation costs.

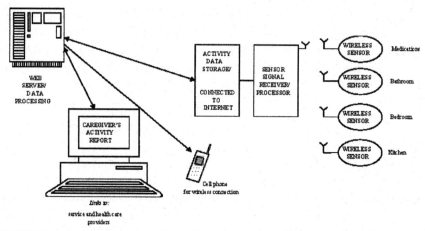

FIGURE 9.1 Behavioral monitoring system.

WEB-BASED REMOTE MONITORING SITE

The Web-based remote monitoring site consists of a server that provides a multiportal, secure Web site that can be accessed by caregivers, providers and the older persons themselves. The site receives behavioral data from the in-home data acquisition units and translates them into information on the activities of the monitored person that can be accessed in the form of a report by any device capable of connecting to the Internet. A PIN is used to access the Web site and specific report pages for either a group of clients or an individual. The report may summarize overall activity levels and/or indicate the status of specific activities, including transferring in and out of bed, bathroom use, meal preparation, eating, and use of medication. Each type of activity is represented by a combination of text and icons that can be displayed by mouse clicks to reveal information about the level of activities. By following easy instructions, current information can be compared with previously collected activity data to flag unexpectedly high or low activity values. These comparisons are continuous and automatic, and any deviations from the individual's normal pattern are flagged as potential problems.

In addition to providing information, a Web-based AATAS can be configured to send e-mail and/or signal an e-mail-based pager. Priority alerts to caregivers and providers relating possible serious problems, i.e., an individual not getting out of bed by a given time of day or not leaving the bathroom after a given period of time can be issued automatically via pager and/or phone to designated individuals. As with any exchange of privileged, private information over the Internet, security issues are of prime consideration and, thus, industry standard methods are employed to maximize security, including double encryption, PIN-secured access and means for identifying and certifying the individual computer logging on to the Web site.

USER TERMINALS AND ACTIVITY REPORTS

The user's terminal can be any device capable of accessing Web sites and/or receiving e-mail, e.g., desktops, laptops, PDAs, Web-enabled cell phones. Depending on the needs of family caregivers, health providers, and case managers, various types of information products can be displayed on the Web site. For example, an adult child can access a Web page that displays information for only the single individual for whom she/he is caring. On the other hand, staff in social or health care provider organizations can access a "group report," that provides summary information on several clients. In this application, activity status indicators flag possible problems and more details are obtained at the click of a mouse.

An example of Web site-based activity reports is provided in Figure 9.2, which is a screen shot of a group report. This figure shows a screen shot of a Web site from the Living Independently system "E-Care Assistant." This is a group report showing the activity status of seven seniors in an independent living apartment house at about 9:00 A.M. . Green, yellow and red are used on the Web page to convey information about the status of the monitored activities for each individual. Green indicates that "all in order—no need to check in with the person," yellow indicates a "possible problem—monitor closely," and red signals a "likely problem—call or check in as soon as possible." Though this figure is reproduced in grayscale, it is still possible to see the text designations corresponding to the colored indicators. A case manager or health provider can use her/his mouse to click on "see details" in order to access an activity report for an individual with a non green status indicator.

PAST, PRESENT AND FUTURE

The first applications of a nonobtrusive behavioral monitoring system were developed in the early 1990s, and by 1994 several independent

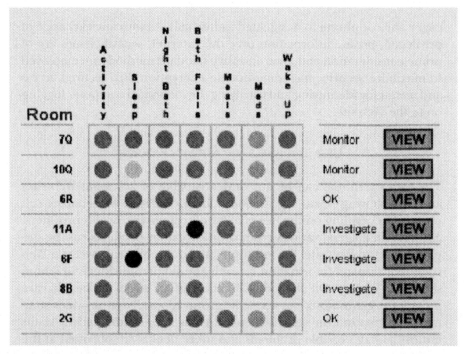

FIGURE 9.2 Group report Web site.

groups had begun to test AATAS prototypes. Notable among these were Celler, Hesketh, Earnshaw, and Islar (1994) in Australia, Tamura, Fujimoto, Moramoto, Haung, Sattaki, and colleagues (1995) in Japan, and Kutzik and Glascock (1994) in the USA. Today there are dozens of projects focused on nonobtrusive monitoring of everyday behavior among the elderly in the U.K., Germany, The Netherlands, Japan, the United States, and Australia. Currently the majority of these projects are in a testing and development phase, but several commercially available systems have appeared on the market. In North America, in addition to Living Independently, Vigil Inc. provides products for the nursing home market, and Home Data Source for the in-home market. Under development are similar systems at the University of Virginia ("MARC"), Honeywell, Inc ("ILSA"), Georgia Tech ("Aware House"), and MIT ("House_n").

While a comprehensive review of different projects is beyond the scope of this chapter, it is informative to briefly compare their designs. All AATAS approaches have a common set of underlying objectives: 1) collecting behavioral data by means of a network of monitors in the home environment; 2) storing and analyzing these data in order to detect changes in behavior over time; and 3) taking automated actions on the basis of this information. However, there are significant differences among the various systems in the use of technology to achieve these objectives.

The first major conceptual distinction is between systems employing minimalist technology and those employing a much more extensive and sophisticated technology. A minimalist approach entails the design and use of the simplest system possible—simple to install, simple to operate, relatively low-level smartness, and the use of available off-the-shelf devices that can be employed without modifications. The converse is a system in which sophisticated, specially designed computer hardware and software are used along with sensor hardware employing multiple modalities of data collection (motion, vibration, computerized visual and audio processing). Technologically complex systems often employ extremely sophisticated artificial intelligence in order to deduce the state of the monitored individual from their footsteps and even gestures.

The second major conceptual distinction is between need-driven and technology-driven development. The need-driven approach is widely discussed in engineering and human factors literatures (Hypponen, 1998) and proceeds from a concrete analysis of the specific needs of individuals. Need-driven AATAS research and development starts with the needs of older people to live safely and independently in their homes for as long as possible and seeks appropriate technology to meet these needs. In contrast, technology-driven development starts with the technology and seeks an application for older people. Although this approach can successfully meet the needs of older individuals, it often results in what we term the "jacuzzi syndrome": the use of technology just because it is available. The availability of sophisticated artificial intelligence software and advanced voice-activated hardware does not necessarily mean that it should be employed in an AATAS.

The third distinction is between a technological presence that is nonobtrusive and one that is much more visible and that requires a high degree of conscious interaction by the older person. In a system designed to be as nonobtrusive as possible, the monitored older person need not consciously interact with the AATAS in any way, but just continue her/his daily routine as if the system were not there. A slightly more obtrusive system requires the older person to utilize a specific medication holder or to respond to an automated phone call. In contrast, a much more obtrusive system requires the older person to interact with the system in numerous ways during the course of the day, e.g., a talking stove, talking medicine cabinet, a door that does not open until you hear and acknowledge a reminder as to what time of day it is. An example of an extremely obtrusive system is found in the Matshusta Koriel-Sincere "smart" nursing home in Japan where elders are expected to talk to a wired teddy bear that records not only their responses but the time it takes for the individual to answer the questions (Lytle, 2002).

The final distinction is between low- versus high-cost systems. While it may seem inordinately American to discuss market price, it is likely that cost will be a significant determinant of when and how AATAS will be commercialized. Simple nonobtrusive systems based on existing technology will have a lower cost structure than systems built on "smart-house" platforms. Of course, costs for even the simplest system could be very high depending on the level of monitoring employed and the amount of intervention desired. However, it appears that costs for a relatively simple system will be comparable to a cell phone, alarm system, or cable television—two to three dollars per day.

PARALLEL DEVELOPMENTS

At the risk of oversimplification, the technological features underlying AATAS are the result of an extension and integration of three source technologies: personal emergency response systems (PERS); telemedicine, especially physiological process telemetry; and "smart house" technologies. In order to understand the current developments of AATAS, it is useful to briefly review these antecedent technologies.

Personal emergency response systems (PERS) emerged as a leading-edge technology to assist frail, at-risk older persons in the 1970s. This technology most often uses a pendant to trigger a small radio transmitter that sends a signal to an emergency response center. In 1978, Swedish TeleLarm deployed the "help phone" along with the portable call button, allowing the older person to call an emergency response center while at the same time enabling persons at the remote monitoring center to "listen in" on the older person by means of an extra-sensitive speaker phone capable of hearing voice data throughout the living unit (Stenberg, 1992).

There was a proliferation of PERS technologies in the 1980s with wireless call buttons and two-way speaker phones in Europe, North America, and Japan resulting in well-articulated support service systems and hundreds of thousands of subscribers by 1991 (Dibner, 1992). LifeLine, perhaps the best known of these products in the United States, had, by 1997, over 450,000 subscribers, who, for a monthly fee, could with the push of a button call a remote monitoring station for help as well as carry on a two-way speaker phone conversation (National Association of Small Business Investment Companies, 2003). Research has shown that both PERS users and their families experience a greater sense of personal security and might even have a decreased likelihood of unscheduled hospital admissions and emergency room visits (Roush, Teasdale, Murphy, & Kirk, 1994). Despite a fairly high rate of nonemergency "false alarms" and the need for a sizeable staff of round the clock operators to receive the phone call, these services are sufficiently cost effective (profitable) to support an expanding market of both individual and institutional subscribers.

Telemedicine is the second technology underlying AATAS and can be broadly defined as using telecommunication technology to deliver health services to remote patients and/or to facilitate information exchange among physicians, health specialists and patients to enhance treatment (Bashshur, 1997). For further information on this topic see the chapter by Tran in this volume. Contemporary telemedicine systems use two-way audio, video and data exchange typically mediated by networked computers. These systems provide means for linking provider and patients for a remote "check up" or diagnostic interview, provide educational or training information through interactive conferencing, or provide health professionals with a means of sharing patient information whether it is in the form of images, words, or numbers.

The transmission of diagnostic image data via closed-circuit television dates from the mid 1970s, and real time video teleconferencing was in place by the mid 1980s using microwave links (Gitlin, 1997). However, automatic acquisition and transmission of physiological data (such as electrocardiograms, respiration, and blood pressure) was not widely used until the advent of dial-up data transfer using laptop computers in the 1990s. Telemetric applications were developed in the United States primarily for military battlefield use and included a variety of appliances to be worn by soldiers that provided real-time remote monitoring of their vital signs (Jones & Satava, 1997). At approximately the same time, Japanese researchers developed a variety of civilian applications for collecting data such as heart rate, blood pressure, respiration, hydration, and weight in the home environment (Togawa, 1992). Of particular note is the work of Alyfuku and Hiruta (1994) on nonobtrusive means for collecting and analyzing physiological data by embedding detectors in the home environment. In this application, an exercise bike measures and records a variety of physiological performance data including heart rate and calorie consumption, a bathtub becomes a means of measuring at-rest heart rate, and a specially equipped toilet becomes a means of analyzing urine and stool samples for possible pathological problems. This embedding of monitoring devices in the home environment and the use of everyday behaviors to provide the context of measurement anticipates several core features of contemporary AATAS applications.

Home automation technologies, the development of which also date from the 1970s, are the third technology underlying AATAS. Home automation entails the control of appliances and environmental systems in a house by means of remote control units, either directly actuated by the user or programmed by means of a computer. By the mid 1980s, it was possible to control lights, appliances, heating, and cooling by remote control unit communication protocols that sent signals through the existing power lines within the building, thereby requiring minimal, if any, retrofitting (Driscoll, 2002). By the mid 1990s, X-10, an industry leader in inexpensive home automation controllers, had sold millions of devices in North America and Europe. While most consumers of home automation products used a "dumb" computerless network of remote controls, a Web-based virtual community of hobbyists and developers working on ways to control one's house by means of a personal computer had sprung up by 1996. Notable were several interest groups especially concerned with using home automation to extend the functioning of handicapped individuals in their homes as well as the use of remote Web sites to monitor and control home automation devices.

The most extensive use of the home automation approach is found in a "smart house." The smart house approach, whether developed in the U.S., Europe, or Japan, relies on the use of computer-driven integration of home automation control systems in which the system itself makes decisions anticipating the desires and needs of the user. Such systems use a combination of controls and sensor arrays to recognize the patterns of motion, appliance use, and activities of the occupants, and to carry out reactions to them. Thus an occupant may wake in the morning, trigger a series of motion detectors, and the coffee maker could turn on automatically.

In its early embodiments, smart house designs catered to well heeled technology enthusiasts who wished to dim their lights, play mood music, draw their drapes, and start their Jacuzzi remotely via their cell phones. However, the potential of intelligent, interactive control systems in the homes of persons with mobility problems and/or cognitive disabilities intrigued both researchers and practitioners. A hallway that automatically lights a path from the bedroom to the bathroom may be a small convenience to a fully mobile individual, but it is a matter of both safety and great convenience to a person in a wheel chair. Similarly, a system that ensures that the ambient temperature stays within a healthful range may be a luxury to a healthy person but a lifesaver to a frail old person with an impaired sense of temperature.

With the development of increasingly sophisticated ubiquitous computing systems in the mid to late 1990s, it became feasible for systems to respond to very subtle actions by the occupants ranging from changes in gait, to gestures, to voice commands. These technical improvements coupled with a growing interest in how to use smart house technology to help impaired persons remain safe and independent have led to an emerging vision of the smart house, which plays an active role in the lives of frail elderly occupants by assuming functions traditionally provided by human caregivers. These systems could be programmed to remind the monitored individuals to turn off the stove or take their medication, query them if they are alright and, if need be, call for help if there appears to be an emergency, such as a person falling and being unable to get up.

BUNDLING: ACHIEVING TELECARE'S FULL POTENTIAL

Thus, at the turn of the 21st century there were four distinct "product lines" that utilized a very similar technology: personal emergency response systems; telemedicine; home automation; and AATAS. Each of these "monitoring technologies" is currently a stand-alone application that targets a specific need of a particular population, e.g., PERS for emergency response for at-risk individuals. However, it is the integration of these four "product lines" that will allow for the full potential of the monitoring technology to be achieved and lead to what we refer to as "telecare." It is difficult to predict the precise "look" of telecare, but it will definitely include components that are currently part of each of the four existing monitoring technologies. The actual mix will depend on the particular needs of the client/customer/patient, but the flexibility of the underlying microprocessor technology of each of the existing "product lines" should result in a telecare system that is able to conform easily and economically to a wide variety of applications.

In all likelihood, though, there will be a core structure to an integrated telecare system on which the various applications will be based. At the heart of this core will be the Internet because currently the Internet is the only economical way to send, store, and retrieve the immense amount of data and information that would be produced by such an integrated system. Therefore, the development of an Internet platform that is flexible enough to allow the integration of the four monitoring technologies is essential. This platform does not necessarily need to employ sophisticated artificial intelligence, but it will need to be both robust and simple. In other words, it must be able to process, almost instantaneously, huge amounts of data while at the same time being able to present information in an easily understood and completely reliable form.

Also essential to any integrated telecare system will be a set of core monitoring features, along with the capacity for the system to respond to emergencies and send reminders and alerts. Although the inherent flexibility of the system will allow for a multitude of monitoring features, some combination of environmental, security, behavioral, and physiological monitoring will be included in the core of most, if not all, systems. It is easy to envision a telecare system that monitors the smoke detectors in a residence, notifies caregivers if the ambient temperature in the residence is dangerously high or low, buzzes if the front door is not locked, and sends an alert if there is a danger of water overflowing from the bathtub. Once the appropriate platform is developed, these environmental features can be readily combined with a burglar alarm system that can provide an even higher level of security.

Security will be further enhanced by the inclusion of the monitoring of a core set of behavioral activities. This core set will probably include whether an individual is up and around, bathroom or toilet use, meal preparation, and the taking of medication, but, as discussed above, other activities can be included depending on the individual's particular needs. Again, depending on need, physiological measures will be included in a basic telecare system. The most typical measures to be included will be blood pressure, weight, and blood sugar level, but as telemedicine applications become more reliable, other health indicators can and will be included.

An integrated telecare system will also include both active and passive emergency response capabilities. The system will provide active emergency response similar to that provided today by PERS through the use of some type of call button. In addition, the system will provide passive emergency response by notifying caregivers if a specific activity has gone unrecorded beyond a predetermined threshold period, e.g., an individual has been in the bathroom beyond the threshold and therefore may have fallen. Finally, a fully developed and bundled system will allow for the provision of a series of reminders. These may include reminders to lock the door when leaving the residence, to take medication, to turn off the stove, and even to check in with a caregiver. The form, frequency, and number of these reminders will depend on individual need, but the capacity will be included in the core of the basic telecare system.

When will such a system be available? This is a difficult question to answer, not from a technological perspective because the technology exists today to create a bundled telecare system, but from a marketing perspective. It is obvious that there is a potential market for such a system: there are currently 30 million Americans over the age of 65 living alone and 22 million households providing part-time care for many of these individuals. There are, therefore, a sufficient number of individuals who could benefit from a telecare system, but the questions as to who will develop such a system, who will use such a system, and who will pay for such a system remain to be answered.

ACKNOWLEDGMENTS

David M. Kutzik is Associate Professor of Sociology and Associate Director, Center for Applied Neurogerontology, Drexel University, Philadelphia, Pennsylvania. Anthony P. Glascock is affiliated with the Department of Culture and Communication, Drexel University, Philadelphia, Pennsylvania.

REFERENCES

Alyfuku, K., & Hiruta, Y. (1994). Networked health care and monitoring system, U.S. Patent # 5,410,471. Retrieved May 2003 from patft.uspto.gov/.

Bashshur, R. (1997). Telemedicine and the health care system. In R. Bashshur, J. Sanders, & G. Shannon, (Eds.), *Telemedicine theory and practice.* Springfield, MA: Charles C Thomas, Ltd.

Celler, B., Hesketh, T., Earnshaw, W., & Ilsar, E. (1994). An instrumentation system for the remote monitoring of changes in functional health status of the elderly at home. *Proceedings of the IEEE Engineering in Medicine and Biology Society, 16*(2), 908.

Dibner, A. (1992). Introduction. In A. Dibner (Ed.), *Personal response systems.* Binghamton, NY: Haworth Press.

Driscoll, E. (2002). The history of X-10. Retrieved June 2003 from home.planet. nl/~lhendrix/x10_history.htm

Gitlin, J. (1997). Teleradiology. In R. Bashshur, J. Sanders, & G. Shannon, (Eds.), *Telemedicine theory and practice.* Springfield, MA: Charles C Thomas, Ltd.

Glascock, A., & Kutzik, D. (2000). Behavioral telemedicine: A new approach to the continuous nonintrusive monitoring of activities of daily living. *Telemedicine, 6*(1), 33–44.

Hypponen, M. (1998). Activity theory as the basis for design for all. *Proceedings of the 3rd TIDE Congress.* Retrieved July 2003 from www.stakes.fi/tide-cong/213hyppo.htm

Jones, S., & Satava, R. (1997). Battlefield telemedicine: The next generation. In R. Bashshur, J. Sanders, & G. Shannon, (Eds.), *Telemedicine theory and practice.* Springfield, MA: Charles C Thomas, Ltd. .

Kutzik, D., & Glascock, A. (1994). *GeMS: Passive microprocessor based case monitoring-intervention system for selected activities of daily living.* In Proceedings of the International Conference on Assistive Technology.

Lytle, J. (2002). Robot care bears for the elderly. Retrieved July 2003 from news.bbc.co.uk/1/hi/sci/tech/1829021.stm

National Association of Small Business Investment Companies (NASBIC) News (2003). *Success stories: Lifeline.* Retrieved June 2003 from www.nasbic.org/success/stories/lifeline.cfm

Roush, R., Teasdale, T., Murphy, J., & Kirk, M. (1994). Impact of a personal emergency response system on hospital utilization by community residing adults. *Journal of the American Geriatrics Society, 42*(11), SA 76.

Stenberg, B. (1992). The Swedish model of social alarm systems for care of the elderly. In A. Dibner (Ed.), *Personal response systems: An international report of a new home care service.* Binghamton, NY: Haworth Press.

Tamura, T., Fujimoto, T., Moramoto, H., Haung, J., Sattaki, H., & Togawa, T. (1995). The design of an ambulatory physical activity monitor and its application to the daily activity of the elderly. *Proceedings of the IEEE Engineering in Medicine and Biology Society, 17*(2), 1591.

Togawa, T. (1992). Physiological monitoring techniques for home health care. *Biomedical Sciences and Instrumentation, 28,* 105–110.

10

Home, Safe Home: Household and Safety Assistive Technology

Mary Hamil Parker and
Dory Sabata

OVERVIEW

Today's elderly can choose from various housing environments that meet their living and functional needs. This chapter will discuss how technology can be used to enhance these living environments. New technology applications and housing alternatives incorporating universal design and tailored to facilitating aging in place will have a significant impact for the aging baby-boom generation.

Independent community and institutional housing settings provide for different needs and have different requirements with regard to home safety. As noted in the previous chapter, assistive technology serves three major purposes relevant to home safety: 1) detecting unsafe situations or emergencies, 2) facilitating independence and functional performance, and 3) supporting caregivers by facilitating provision of personal care. The single common requirement is that the technology must provide a living environment that accommodates and supports the functional capacities of the residents. Assistive technologies must provide support for individuals' cognitive, perceptual, sensory, and physical capacities; and thereby prevent, mitigate, or compensate for declines resulting from disease or the aging process.

Falls and fire are the most important safety concerns in all housing environments. Falls are the leading cause of injury to older adults in the U.S. Hip fractures, head injury, poisoning by carbon monoxide, and burns are the most common household injuries among older adults (CDC, 2002). Assistive technology and home modifications are important to a multidimensional approach to fall prevention (Rubenstein & Josephson, 2002). Features of the housing environment, e.g., stairs, grab bars, handrails, and lighting can contribute to safety by reducing the potential for loss of balance and falls.

Discussions of home safety often focus exclusively on reducing home hazards—detection of smoke, heat, or carbon-monoxide—using passive sensors that have alarms or flashing lights. In the last 10 years, as communications technology has become wireless and digital, home safety and security equipment is more readily available and easier to install. Smoke detectors and carbon-monoxide detectors can be purchased in supermarkets and drugstores. Home security systems, ranging from outdoor lights to alarms, are available as off-the-shelf, wireless technology at hardware and electronics stores in neighborhood shopping centers. As this chapter demonstrates, this same technology is being adapted and enhanced to provide more sophisticated services to address the safety and personal care needs of frail elderly.

COMMUNITY RESIDENCE

It is important to recognize that older adults reside in diverse living environments, including single-family homes and apartments, congregate senior housing, assisted living, and retirement communities. Many elders have lived in the same single-family home and community for over 30 years. The collective aging of groups of older residents has contributed to the creation of neighborhoods called NORCs (naturally occurring retirement communities). NORCs have developed in commercial apartment developments in many areas, creating rental NORCs, particularly if rent controls have encouraged long-term residence of retirees.

Often older housing requires renovation to adequately meet the needs of aged residents. Most older rental units have not been renovated to accommodate the changed needs of elderly tenants. As a result, living in older buildings involves several safety challenges to residents with reduced physical capabilities. Some may find themselves imprisoned in multistory homes and "walk-up" apartments, which they rarely leave because of the physical demands of negotiating staircases.

The National Older Adult Housing Survey of the National Association of Home Builders (NAHB, 2002) documented important residential and community features for persons age 65 and older. The most desired feature mentioned by the elderly who were surveyed was lower crime rates; other features mentioned were less home maintenance effort and cost, a pleasant climate, lower cost of living, home safety features like security alarms, and proximity to health care. Over half of all respondents did not have any home modifications related to health, (e.g., grab bars in the tub/shower and around the toilet, hand-held shower nozzles, easy to reach shelving, or audible or visual strobe light alarm systems).

In a reduction of the trend for seniors to move to a warmer climate, about two-thirds of builders in the 2002 NAHB survey reported that their customers were relocating from the same community or the same state. Nearly half of these buyers indicated a desire to be closer to children, grandchildren, and family. Builders are developing recreational retirement communities restricted to residents age 50 and older. Three out of four single-family homes for seniors started during 2002 were one-story and more than half had strategically placed streetlights, intercoms or entrance phones, and home security systems. Indicative of today's seniors' technological savvy, nearly 70 percent of new communities had high-speed Internet service.

In many communities there is a zoning trend toward requiring design in all new residential construction to accommodate mobility and other impairments. These "universal design" features have numerous home safety benefits for all ages. No-step, at grade entrances reduce the chance of falls, while increasing the ability of elderly persons and those with mobility impairments to safely and easily enter and exit the home, even if using a walker or wheelchair. Widening of doorways and hallways makes it easier for people using mobility aides to safely navigate within the home. The ability to operate doors is enhanced by levers instead of doorknobs. Single-lever controls on kitchen and lavatory faucets are easier to operate and make adjustments of water temperature and volume simple for everyone. Electrical outlets located several feet up the wall are more reachable by those who may have trouble bending or reaching.

Creating a safe living environment requires reduced glare and sufficient ambient and task lighting to compensate for age-related vision changes. Lighting should be provided in a variety of locations and at different levels to reduce glare and decrease shadows. Light switches should be located at the entrance to each room to permit sufficient illumination for the older resident to safely enter and move about. A useful alternative to the standard light switch is voice- or noise- (clapping) activated switches (Center for Universal Design, 2003).

Such adaptations particularly benefit people with limited mobility, yet all members of a household, young and old, benefit from safer homes that facilitate daily activities. Housing built or renovated using universal design principles can allow families to "age in place" without incurring significant remodeling expenses.

Older homes can be modified to incorporate universal design features after a comprehensive assessment to determine how to meet the individual needs of residents and the best types of AT for that person. However planning and making these changes, including the selection of adaptive equipment, can be intimidating for the average older consumer. Many people on fixed incomes may fear the cost, while many localities lack trained, responsible, knowledgeable modification providers.

To facilitate access to adaptive home modification, Extended Home Living Services, a private construction firm in Wheeling, Illinois, has developed a computerized system for assessing home modification needs under a grant from the National Institute on Aging. This Comprehensive Assessment and Solutions Process for Aging Residents (CASPAR) enables nonspecialists in home modification to collect information about needs from the elderly consumer and then send this data to specialists in home modification who identify problems and design individualized solutions. CASPAR has been shown to have both inter-rater reliability in the measurement process and criterion validity in the assessment process (Sanford, 2002).

HOME SAFETY ADAPTATIONS FOR DEMENTIA CAREGIVING

Little research has been done to determine the effect of environmental modifications on the way people with cognitive impairments interact with their living environments and how these might reduce the burden of caregiving. Calkins and Namazi (1991) surveyed a purposive sample of 59 Alzheimer's support group participants and family members of dementia patients placed in nursing homes to determine what changes they had made while caregiving in the home to deal with wandering, incontinence, safety, independence, and reduction of havoc and confusion. All 59 had made at least one environmental change, most frequently from concern for the safety of the person with dementia. Eighty-five percent of the modifications helped caregivers and 77% benefited the person with dementia. Wandering was the most frequently mentioned problem (69%) leading to

46 modifications (including adding a deadbolt or chain lock, disguising or blocking the door, or locking the screen door); 73% were reported to work well. In dealing with safety and independence, 63% had made at least one modification to the bathroom, and 56% made modifications to the kitchen. There were 62 bathroom modifications, and 91% were reported to work well, (included removing medicines, installing a shower or tub chair, adding grab bars to toilet or tub, adding a nonskid tub mat, and installing a hand-held shower head). Of the 95 kitchen modifications, 76% were reported to work well (included unplugging appliances and removing equipment, installing a separate power switch for the stove, and placing signs indicating potential hazards). Other room modifications included removal of long electrical cords, adding bed rails, and putting a gate in front of the stairs. Living and dining rooms had 59 changes with 85% reported to be working well. Bedrooms had 67 changes, with 79% reported to be working well. There were 27 changes to stairs, with 78% working well (Calkins & Namazi, 1991).

Senior Housing and Supportive Living Arrangements

The aging of America has prompted the development of specialized senior housing and commercial marketing of a wide variety of living arrangements that offer supportive and nursing care. Congregate senior housing for independent, low- and moderate-income elderly has been developed under federal requirements of the U.S. Department of Housing and Urban Development and the Farmers Home Administration, U.S. Department of Agriculture. Federally subsidized senior housing is mandated to provide safety features like grab bars and emergency pull cords in the bathroom; pull cords may be in the bedroom or living room as well. Older federally subsidized senior housing, intended for "independent well elderly," did not contemplate "aging in place," and unless renovated they lack accommodations for handicapped individuals. To reduce construction costs, some newer senior buildings do not provide elevators, congregate dining, social areas, or space for medical and other services.

The accessibility requirements of the Fair Housing Act apply to buildings with five or more units built for first occupancy after March 13, 1991. These buildings must have 5%, or at least one unit, whichever is greater, accessible for persons with mobility impairments in accordance with the Uniform Federal Accessibility Standards (UFAS), and the Architectural Barriers Act, 42 U.S.C. 4151–4157. An additional 2% of units, or at least one unit, must be equipped for persons with hearing or visual disabilities and have strobe flashing and audible alarms (www.hud.gov/offices/fheo/disabilities/accessibilityR.cfm).

Continuing Care Retirement Communities (CCRCs) offer several levels of care on the same campus or in the same building—independent apartments or freestanding cottages, an assisted living/supported housing unit, a nursing facility, and sometimes a special-care dementia unit. People pay an entrance fee and monthly charges, which may be fixed or based upon services used, and are guaranteed care for the remainder of their lives. There are currently approximately 1,200 such facilities in the U.S. (Scanlon & Layton, 1997).

Assisted living is the fastest growing residential option; there are more than 28,000 such facilities in the U.S. (NCAL, 1998). They are attractive due to their provision of services and features such as meal preparation (76%), personal assistance (65%), housekeeping (64%), health services (50%), social activities (43%), laundry (42%), and transportation (32%) (NAHB 2002).

Currently, there are no federal regulatory requirements for the types of care provided in independent retirement housing and assisted living facilities, aside from basic zoning and fire safety and similar regulations, unless part of the facility is certified for Medicare/Medicaid. However, some states have established oversight mechanisms for assisted living facilities, particularly those that have Alzheimer's disease or dementia units. Also, the U.S. Senate Special Committee on Aging encouraged assisted living stakeholders (providers, consumers, and other interested national groups) to develop recommendations for Committee consideration (Assisted Living Workgroup, 2003).

An estimated 1. 6 million people live in the 18,000 nursing homes in the United States (NCHS, 1999). Regulations for nursing facilities certified to receive Medicare/Medicaid payments assure basic fire safety measures such as sprinklers and fire/emergency safety plans. Older nursing homes were constructed like hospitals with long corridors and central nursing stations. Newer and remodeled facilities are designed with features to create a more residential/homelike environment, with smaller "neighborhood" units providing dining and social areas for small groups of residents, shorter and wider hallways, central living/recreational spaces and access to outdoor sitting areas. Some facilities provide pets and gardens for a "homelike" environment. Standards require adequate fire safety, emergency plans and equipment, and six hours of fire safety training for staff annually, to protect residents and provide safe evacuation.

ASSISTIVE TECHNOLOGIES TO
SUPPORT INDEPENDENT LIVING

Assistive technology that can increase safety, while preserving independence for the frail elderly, is becoming commercially available. A growing number of companies are beginning to market sophisticated passive and active monitoring systems.

PERSONAL RESPONSE SYSTEMS (PERS)

The most established AT home safety application is the Personal Emergency Response System (PERS). The first of these systems was developed in the 1970s by Lifeline Systems, Inc., based upon research in a Massachusetts nursing facility, and now is used by millions of older people in the United States. Lifeline's success fostered development of similar systems and services by other companies.

PERSs are intended to provide access to emergency assistance, 24 hours a day, 7 days a week, 365 days a year, to help people who fall and are unable to get up, or who have another medical emergency such as a heart attack. Data indicate that the risk of being found "down or dead" increases with age, from 3 per 1000 for people age 60–64 to 123 per 1000 for people age 85 and older living alone, with a 23% risk of death for those who cannot get up (Gurley, Lum, Sande, Lo, & Katz, 1996). PERSs originally required a user to press an alarm button and send the signal over a nearby telephone line. Microchips and digital and wireless communications technologies have enabled the development of wireless PERSs. One commercially available system can detect if a user has fallen to the floor and others now use wireless video cameras.

A study by Teasdale and Roush (2001) used Lifeline to see if users felt more secure with the technology. The study used a randomized block sampling method designed to select by gender, age 70 or over, living alone, at risk for fall, recent surgery, and cardiology or pulmonary diagnosis. Of 269 participants, 90 received a PERS for 12 months; 88 received a PERS for 6 months, which was then discontinued, and 89 in the control group did not receive a PERS. All participants received bimonthly phone calls for one year to collect reports of their perception of security with and without a PERS, and responses on ADL-IADL, SF-36, and other psychometric measures. All users reported a greater sense of security during their PERS use (p = 0.0001). The study dropout-rate tripled in subjects asked to give up the device for 6 months. The 12-month users improved in vitality, role-emotional, and mental health SF-36 scores (all $p < 0.005$). Vitality and mental health significantly improved, compared with nonusers. The results indicate that PERS users perceive support that positively affects their ability to function.

Cueing and reminding for medications and appointments have been added to most commercially available PERS services to provide additional support for older adults with the types of cognitive changes discussed in a previous chapter by Mayhorn, Rogers, and Fisk. Sunrise Corporation, a major provider of assisted living, has introduced "Lifeline With Reminders" as a new marketing initiative for their home care and other services, not only providing reminders for residents to take medications and go to appointments, but also allowing families to remotely record up to six personal family voice reminder messages and deliver them at selected times.

UNIVERSAL DESIGN AND SMART HOME TECHNOLOGY

As people begin to experience difficulties with their daily activities, they are at increased risk for accidents. Assistive technologies that compensate for changes in vision, hearing, mobility, and acuity of senses can enhance home safety. These passive monitors can signal the person about a hazard—for example a stove or appliance left on or water running—by sounding an alarm or flashing a light. They can also send a notification of the danger to a remote location for emergency responders or family. Privately and publicly funded research continues to develop new approaches, but none are yet widely available in the marketplace, and there are many issues about the local availability and cost of such systems.

INTELLIGENT BUILDING TECHNOLOGY

Intelligent building technology, sometimes referred to as "smart" housing, can support the activities of people with physical disabilities and aging people by reducing the physical and cognitive demands in the environment. The early example design houses built by the National Association of Home Builders and Aware House at the Georgia Institute of Technology were intended as technology showcases, not residences, and used hard wiring to support innovations to control heating/cooling, lights, windows, and doors. However, the cost of this technology was out of reach for many consumers since it was expensive and sometimes impossible to add to existing housing. All this has changed with the development of wireless technology, which uses radio signals and the existing wiring to send signals throughout the home, making it possible and affordable for people with disabilities and other family members to take advantage of new assistive and adaptive technology.

FUTURE HOME

A striking illustration of the evolution of assistive technology from hard wired to wireless is provided by Future Home, the home of David Ward, a quadriplegic as a result of a spinal cord injury. A 135-year-old tavern in Jarretsville, Maryland, listed on the Maryland Historic Registry, the Future Home building was renovated to provide a showcase of universal design for independent living for people with disabilities and those who want to age in place. The addition of technology enables Mr. Ward, who lives with a relative and a personal assistant, to carry on daily activities advocating for disability rights in Maryland and function independently, using assistive devices and a computer.

The rehabilitation of Future Home in 1990 used commercially available products and systems, adapting or enhancing them to allow Mr. Ward to control his environment (e.g., turning lights on and off; identifying visitors at the door and allowing entrance to the home; controlling heating/cooling; turning on a fan, or summoning assistance) using his voice, breath, and the limited use of one arm in a brace. This technology cost an estimated $60,000, principally for the installation of wiring in the walls (hard wiring) and specialized software.

However, after seven years, Ward found that many of the products used were no longer available to the consumer, even though they functioned well at Future Home. Mr. Ward wanted to preserve Future Home's function as a living showcase, and to take advantage of the greater flexibility and range of activities offered by changes in computer and digital technology. So in 2002, he upgraded using wireless technology at an estimated cost of $8,500. A simple touch keypad and pointer replaced most of the functions handled by the earlier hard-wired technology and specially programmed software. This illustrates how off-the-shelf technology and cutting-edge assistive technology have become much more affordable for individuals who need it most, and for the average consumer (Ward & Parker, 2002).

Older persons responding to the NAHB survey had concerns about cost, maintenance, safety, and access to health care. Their principle concern was the cost for adaptation of existing housing and the maintenance of the AT. Technology for home safety must address security and responsiveness of safety monitoring services, as well as the intersection of home technologies with health care monitoring. Telemedicine and telerehabilitation have increased access to medical oversight in the home, but the uninsured costs are prohibitive for most consumers.

A survey of 176 PERS or other alarm users, with a mean age of 76 years, indicated that 77% were interested in automatic fall detection, 68% were interested in lifestyle monitoring, 57% in telemedicine, and 46% in videoconferencing (Brownsell, Bradley, Bragg, Catlin, & Carlier, 2000). The commercial potential of these and other assistive technology applications in the home have been recognized by U.S. businesses and are being supported and encouraged by government funding agencies.

ASSISTIVE TECHNOLOGY IN THE SUPPORTIVE AND LONG TERM CARE ENVIRONMENT

Safety is a primary concern in living environments for groups of frail, disabled, or demented elderly. Assisted living and nursing facilities use assistive technology in units specially designed to meet the needs of people with Alzheimer's disease and other dementias and to prevent them from exiting the unit unescorted. Some facilities are exploring ways to use assistive technology to supplement direct staff supervision, while assuring resident safety and fostering independent functioning.

ASSISTED LIVING USE OF UNIVERSAL DESIGN AND TECHNOLOGY

Elite Care, an assisted living company located in Oregon, has created Oatfield Estates, Extended Family Residences™, a state-licensed housing project using concepts of universal design and information from research about optimal long-term care environments (Donahue, 2001; Berck, 2001). The facility is located in an established suburban neighborhood to provide residents the benefit of surrounding community facilities. In both form and scale, buildings are family-style residences for up to fifteen people. Private rooms, with the resident's own furniture, memorabilia, and choice of decoration, open onto large common spaces, such as a "country kitchen," activity room, and great room. Short hallways make it easy for residents to access common spaces.

While many upscale senior living facilities offer such amenities, what is unique is the use of "smart home" technology to assist residents and staff. Each resident wears a badge the size of a credit card that sends an infrared signal to embedded sensors in ceilings and walls. The badge also serves as an individual room key. The passive monitoring sensors indicate when residents are in their rooms. Other sensors are activated to prevent the stove or other appliances from being turned on if a cognitively impaired resident enters the kitchen alone. There is a computer in each resident's room, and access to the Internet and e-mail enhances their social connections. In the future, individual medical monitoring or voice reminders will assist with daily functioning and provide staff with information about residents to identify health problems. The system software, CARE™ will gather, store and transmit health information using digital technology and the Internet, in real time, while also monitoring the ambient environment, and adjusting heating, cooling, and lighting.

NURSING FACILITIES

A variety of assistive devices can help nursing facilities meet Federal requirements for reduction in the use of physical restraints, while protecting frail residents who are at risk of falling. These sensor alarms are as simple as a cord attached to the resident's clothing that sets off an alarm when the resident stretches it in rising from a chair or bed. These sensor pads, placed in the bed or on the floor beside the bed, send silent alarms to a nursing station when the resident gets up or steps on the floor.

Other devices and video cameras are used to detect abuse or neglect of residents by caregiving staff. Issues of staff and resident privacy arise with application of this monitoring technology. Some states have considered laws that authorize the use of electronic monitoring devices in the room of a nursing home resident for these purposes. These laws would provide a form releasing the nursing facility from civil liability for violation of the privacy rights of the resident receiving surveillance, as well as a consent form for such electronic monitoring and signs that announce the use of such equipment.

THE FUTURE OF HOME SAFETY TECHNOLOGY

The National Institute on Aging (NIA) of the National Institutes of Health, U.S. Department of Health and Human Services, has a new technology and aging initiative. In January 2003 the National Research Council, National Academy of Sciences, held a two-day workshop, with sponsorship from the National Institute on Aging, on technology for adaptive aging, which addressed ways in which technology can be developed and applied to improve the lives of an aging population. A number of nationally recognized experts discussed potential applications of technology to the domains of living environments, health, communication, education and learning, transportation, and employment. A special emphasis was given to the challenges of translating laboratory successes into useful, marketable products and services appropriate for small business innovation research (SBIR) and other grant funding from the National Institutes of Health and other federal agencies. A collection of the papers presented is available from the National Academies Press and can be reviewed at www.nap.edu/aging. The NIA is actively stimulating studies that translate knowledge about aging from basic behavioral and social science research into products and services of benefit to elderly and the systems providing health care, as well as new "use-inspired" basic research in the behavioral and social sciences.

The National Institute of Science and Technology (NIST) and the NIA, have given grants to U.S. researchers and businesses to develop assistive technology systems that would meet some of these needs. Some of the results are described below.

ILSA: HONEYWELL INTERNATIONAL

NIST funded a 2.5-year, $5 million research and development program with Honeywell International to develop a prototype intelligent home automation system, called Independent Life Style Assistant (ILSA). Honeywell has long experience in control systems and home automation and believes that in many cases the needs of the elderly could be served better—and less expensively—by an intelligent, home-based automation system that enables individuals to continue to live safely at home in an assisted environment. ILSA uses components similar to the system described by Kutzik and Glascock in an earlier chapter. The project is being led by Honeywell Laboratories and includes geriatric and gerontological specialists from the University of Minnesota School of

Nursing, United HealthCare Corporation's EverCare Division, and the University of Florida.

When fully implemented, ILSA will integrate a diverse set of passive motion sensors, medication dispensers, medical monitoring devices and "smart" appliances, using automated reasoning and situation assessment based on information about the individual's medical diagnoses and functional assessment. ILSA will collect and analyze these data to determine a person's needs and adapt monitoring to identify and respond to critical situations, provide reminders, and support usual daily activities. For example, the system will identify whether a medication caddy has been opened during the time window when the older person has been reminded to take medications, and if this time window is exceeded and the individual does not take the medication after a specified time, the system will send a notice to a caregiver. User-friendly features such as voice interaction will eliminate the need for elders to "master" the technology. ILSA will assess a situation, understand the elder's immediate needs, and adapt itself to meet those needs. When ILSA determines that outside assistance is needed, it will summon help.

In Phase One, Honeywell tested a prototype of this system containing basic medication and mobility monitoring features. Tests were conducted in four single-family homes in Florida and five independent living community apartments in Minnesota. Data was collected through weekly interviews with clients and their caregivers, as well as extensive data logs generated by the system. For additional information, see www.htc.honeywell.com/projects/ilsa/.

PROACTIVE HEALTH RESEARCH INITIATIVE: INTEL CORPORATION

In April 2002, the Intel Corporation announced its Proactive Health Research initiative (www.intel.com/research/prohealth). The goal is to understand how technology can support individual behaviors that help prevent disease, foster independence, and improve quality of life, as well as the use of technology to meet the growing shortage in home care workers. Initially, the focus is on identifying markers of physical and cognitive decline and the way technologies can help elderly to age in place wherever they are living. This will involve three types of research: 1) ethnographic field research in people's homes to identify their needs through observation and interviews, 2) application of these field results to develop and test prototypes of future home systems that could meet the health needs of an entire multigenerational household, 3) outcome studies of beta prototype systems to determine their effect on targeted needs or desired outcomes. Key collaborators in this project include the University of Washington, the Oregon Health and Science University, the University of Rochester, and the Georgia Institute of Technology.

Part of the Phase One research is a survey of 60 households chosen from across the U.S. with a focus on cognitive impairment, ranging from mild to advanced stages of Alzheimer's disease. To expand this research, in cooperation with the Alzheimer's Association, INTEL has formed the Everyday Technologies for Alzheimer Care (ETAC) consortium to fund more than $1 million of research to develop new models of Alzheimer care using technology to help people with cognitive impairments and their caregivers to live meaningful lives in the community. INTEL's approach to home monitoring involves the placement of radio-frequency tags on clothing or shoes, which interact with sensors in the home. If someone is in the kitchen, sensors in cabinets, the refrigerator, microwave, and dishes would send signals to a computer that would then signal a television set to play a video clip with cueing assistance (Robertson, 2003).

AWARE HOME: GEORGIA INSTITUTE OF TECHNOLOGY

The Aware Home Research Initiative is a collaborative activity of the Georgia Institute of Technology and several corporations, including INTEL, Mitsubishi, Hewlett-Packard, Accenture, and Visteon, as well as federal funding from the National Science Foundation (Sanders, 2002). Aware Home is part of the unique 5,040 square foot Broadband Institute Residential Laboratory. Georgia Tech scientists work with sensing technology to see how they can monitor movements from room to room and record movement and conversations of elderly people, using cameras and microphones embedded in the walls to create a home system which would collect and digitize data to send reports to family members offsite. For example, footsteps can be used to analyze the speed used to walk from room to room or climb stairs and changes in pattern detected by monitoring software. The project is attempting to determine how to design a home that will support the functional independence of elderly residents to postpone or prevent the need to move to assisted living or a nursing facility. To help family members interpret the data produced, Elizabeth Mynatt, a computer science professor at Georgia Tech, is testing a Digital Family Portrait to utilize the sensing information to provide a visual description of person's daily life activities.

CONCLUSION

The speed with which creation of new assistive technologies has been advancing in recent years—becoming smaller, more versatile, and cheaper—bodes well for the future. The number of research activities and the amount of private and public funding addressing these issues has been increasing rapidly. The diverse approaches of these efforts also project an encouraging picture. Soon the elderly living in the community, and those who chose specially designed supportive housing, will have access to various adaptive systems that will effectively help them age safely in their chosen living arrangements.

ACKNOWLEDGMENTS

Mary Hamil Parker is President, MKHP Associates, LLC/Institute for Palliative & Hospice Training, Inc., Alexandria, Virginia. Dory Sabata is Program Specialist, USC Andrus Gerontology Center, National Resource Center on Supportive Housing and Home Modification, Los Angeles, California.

REFERENCES

Assisted Living Workgroup (2003). *Assuring Quality in Assisted Living: Guidelines for Federal and State Policy, State Regulations and Operations. A Report to the U.S. Senate Special Committee on Aging.* Retrieved October 9, 2003 from www.aahsa.org/alw/intro.pdf

Berck, J. (2001, April 5). The wired retirement home. *The New York Times.* Retrieved April 14, 2003 from www.elite-care.com

Centers for Disease Control and Prevention (2001). *Injury Fact Book, National Center for Injury Prevention and Control.* Retrieved April 15, 2003 from www.cdc.gov/ncipc/fact_book/Index.htm

Donahue, B. (2001, May). Byte, byte, against the dying of the light. *The Atlantic Monthly, 287,* 28–30. Retrieved October 9, 2003, from www.theatlantic.com/issues/2001/05/donahue.htm

National Center for Assisted Living (1998). *1998 facts and trends: The assisted living sourcebook.* Washington, DC: National Center for Assisted Living.

National Center on Health Statistics (2002). *National Nursing Home Survey.* Retrieved June 12, 2003 from www.cdc.gov/nchs/about/major/nnhsd/nnhsd.htm

NAHB Research Center (2002). *National Older Adult Housing Survey 2002.* Upper Marlboro, MD: Author.

Robertson, C. (2003). Exploring Technology's Caring Side. *The New York Times, July 20.*

Sanders, J., (2002). There's no place like home. *Research Horizons.* Retrieved April 14, 2003, from www.gtresearchnews.gatech.edu/reshor/rh-f01/

Scanlon, W., & Layton, B. D. (1997). *Report to Congressional requesters: How continuous care retirement communities manage services for the elderly.* Washington, DC: U.S. General Accounting Office.

Teasdale, T. A., & Roush, R. E. (2001, November). *Perception of Safety With and Without a Personal Response System (PRS).* Symposium presentation at the 54th Annual Meeting of the Gerontological Society of America, Chicago, Illinois.

11

Technologies To Facilitate Health and Independent Living in Elderly Populations

Binh Q. Tran

The graying of America and of the global population presents tremendous challenges to society at many levels—social, political, and economical. The current size of the population age 65 and older in the United States is approximately 33 million (12.7% of the U.S. population in 1999); it is projected to be 53 million by 2020, and 77 million by 2040 (U.S. Census Bureau, 2001). While the U.S. population as a whole has tripled in the past 100 years, astonishingly, the elderly population has grown elevenfold over the same period. Clearly, the elderly segment of the U.S. population continues to experience tremendous growth for various reasons ranging from improved health and medical care, to improved living conditions and safety standards, to better overall quality of life.

In the U.S., data from 1994–95 reveal that over half the elderly (52.5%) reported having at least one disability and approximately one-third reported having a severe disability (U.S. Census Bureau, 1997). According to the Census Bureau, over 4.4 million (14%) Americans have difficulty independently performing normal activities of daily living (ADLs) and 6.5 million (21%) have difficulty carrying out instrumental activities of daily living (IADLs). While disabilities may limit one's ability to perform ADLs and/or IADLs, a recent study documents a strong desire by the elderly (over 95%) to age in their own homes, i.e., "age in place" (U.S. Census Bureau, 1997).

Several health factors act to limit independence in elderly populations. A report by the Robert Wood Johnson Foundation (1998) found that at least 100 million Americans, many of them elderly, suffer from chronic diseases. Approximately 25 million of this group are disabled because of their disease and related complications. In *Healthy People 2010,* the U.S. Department of Health & Human Services reported statistics relating to deaths by chronic illness. Cardiovascular disease (31.4%), followed by cancer (23.3%), respiratory diseases (7.8%), and stroke (6.9%), are the leading cause of death among those age 65 and older (U.S. Department of Health & Human Services, 2000). Alone, heart disease, cancer, and stroke account for over 1.1 million deaths annually among those age 65 and older. Heart disease is also the leading cause of disability among older adults. Data suggests that over 12 million Americans are living with coronary heart disease and another 4 million have suffered from an episodic stroke event. In addition, 50 million Americans are estimated to be living with high blood pressure, commonly called "the silent killer" because many sufferers often go undiagnosed (American Heart Association, 2002).

Each year statistics on these and other chronic illnesses continue to rise. With each advancing decade, the prevalence of these diseases increases in the population. It is important to note that while statistics on *individual* chronic illnesses are readily available, data regarding those living with *comorbidities,* are more difficult to obtain. A study by Guralnik, LaCroix, and Everett (1989) conducted for the National Center for Health Statistics reported that the percentage of elderly individuals living with at least two chronic conditions was approximately 25.9% of those surveyed. The study estimated that 14.6% were living with at least three comorbidities.

Furthermore, several aging-related physiologic changes also lead to symptoms that negatively impact quality of life in the elderly. Examples include urinary incontinence, sensory deficits, pressure ulcers, sleep disorders, and nutritional and eating disorders. Exacerbation in any of these may result in loss of independence or, in severe cases, a need for institutionalized care.

GROWTH OF TECHNOLOGIES: RETROSPECTIVE REVIEW

Parallel to the aging phenomena, the world is witnessing a proliferation of technologies. A myriad of emerging technologies, ranging from computing to information to telecommunications to health care technologies, offer tremendous opportunities to benefit elderly individuals and to assist them in their quest to "age in place." Computing and information technologies have experienced rapid expansion within the last decade. The Internet, as we perceive it today, was a nascent technology until the early 1990s. Until then, it was a playground reserved for academics, researchers, the military, and technophiles. When researchers at the National Center for Supercomputing Applications (NCSA) at the University of Illinois at Urbana-Champaign developed a graphic user interface (GUI) program (i.e., Mosaic) to more easily navigate the Internet, the flood gates to this medium were thrown wide open. Today, use of e-mail and the Internet is ubiquitous and has been so infused that the medium is a viable option for conducting commercial transactions.

The health care arena is slowly progressing with regard to adoption of computer and Internet technology for improving access and quality of service for at-home consumers. While electronic transfer of information provides obvious advantages in facilitating communication with patients and consumers as well as enabling health information data collection, issues and barriers affecting widespread adoption of new technologies in health care include provisions for safety, security, confidentiality, and privacy of information that meet standards established by the Health Insurance Portability and Accountability Act (HIPAA).

Simultaneous to the rapid growth in computer and information technologies, a concurrent explosion in telecommunications capabilities has engendered growth in the area of wireless communications. A key example is the ubiquitous use of cellular phones in today's society. Combined, wireless communications and computer/information technologies present exciting opportunities for home health care delivery. These technologies have particular relevance to the fields of telehealth and telemedicine. For one, wireless technologies may serve to benefit those living with chronic diseases as these technologies provide the means for health consultation, for collecting physiologic and other health related information, for ensuring safety and environmental control, for enabling independent living through home automation, and for a host of other possibilities. The rapid ascent of mobile wireless technologies promises to provide the heterogeneous user (i.e., elderly consumer, health practitioner, and caregiver) with the appealing prospect of accessing "information anywhere."

At the HomeCare & Telerehabilitation (HCTR) Technology Center at The Catholic University of America, researchers and engineers have been involved with evaluating and developing technologies for delivery of health care services to the home environment. The proliferation of computer, information, telecommunications, and sensor technologies, often targeted for other markets, has great potential in the field of home health care. A central focus of our work has been the integration of wireless strategies into the future delivery of home health care and more generally to other respects of independent living. Following the findings of the MacArthur Foundation studies on aging (Rowe & Kahn, 1998), the HCTR Technology Center has focused its multifaceted strategy to support successful aging by applying novel and innovative technologies to achieve three goals: 1) avoiding disease, 2) maintaining physical and cognitive function, and 3) lifelong engagement. A conceptual model of the various roles of technology in promoting independent living and successful aging is shown in Figure 11.1.

TECHNOLOGIES FOR AVOIDING DISEASE

As stated previously, a large percentage of the elderly and old-elderly are living with chronic disease or disability, many with comorbidities (Guralnik,

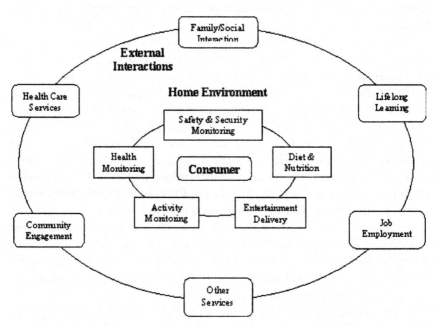

FIGURE 11.1 Planetary model of technology's potential role in "successful aging."

LaCroix, & Everett, 1989). One major challenge to successful aging is the ability *to maintain health and function*. From another perspective, it is the ability *to avoid disease*. Existing and emerging technologies have great promise in redefining the role of home-based care in today's health environment to include disease prevention.

One growing trend in telehealth and home health care delivery is the use of video telephony transmitted over *plain old telephone service* (POTS). POTS-based telephony enables video and audio interactions and communications between at-home patients and remotely located health care professionals. Studies by our group (Buckley, Tran, & Prandoni, 2001; Tran, Kinsella, Winters, Thiel, Prandoni, et al., 1999) have evaluated the performance characteristics of POTS-based telephony for providing health care interactions and support for stroke caregivers from a distance (Tran, Krainak, Lauderdale, & Winters, 2002). We have developed general guidelines for other practitioners on criteria for selection of these technologies for their applications (Tran, Buckley, & Prandoni, 2002). Preliminary data from field studies indicate widespread acceptance and tolerance of technology by elderly patients and caregivers. Videophone communications technology, which provides both audio and visual consultation between caregiver and nurse, was found to have a direct impact on the quality of care and caregiving of stroke patients in the home. Also, somewhat unexpectedly, but perhaps more important, POTS-based telephony was instrumental in providing psychosocial support to reduce caregiver burden, anxiety, isolation, and depression (Buckley, Tran, & Prandoni, 2001).

Emerging technologies beyond video telephony promise to provide a wide range of diagnostic and home monitoring services for management of chronic illness. Telehealth technologies for home monitoring have produced improved outcomes for several chronic illnesses common in older adults. These include heart failure (Fulmer, Feldman, Kim, Carty, Beers, et al., 1999; Kinsella, 1998; Shah, Der, Ruggerio, Heindenreich, & Massie, 1998), respiratory diseases, (Kinsella, 2000a) and diabetes (Gomez, Hernando, Garcia, Del Pozo, Cermeno, et al., 2002; Kinsella, 1999, 2000b). Figure 11.2 shows examples of home health monitoring systems commonly used in monitoring of at-home consumers for improved management of chronic illness. Common system configurations include sensors for measurement of blood pressure, temperature, and heart rate. Specialized systems permit acquisition of electrocardiograms, heart and lung sounds, and blood oxygen levels for those with prevailing cardiac and pulmonary diseases. When connected to in-home

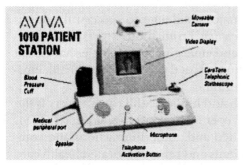 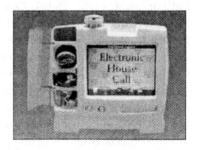

American Telecare-Aviva 1010   CyberCare-EHC 2000

FIGURE 11.2 Examples of two telehealth workstations by American Telecare, Inc. (Eden Prairie, MN) and CyberCare Inc. (Atlanta, GA).

telephone lines, these health monitoring stations serve as a gateway for transmission of health data from the home and often are equipped with video cameras and software for interactive remote consultations.

While the above workstations require users to periodically make physiologic measurements, current research at the HCTR Technology Center (and other laboratories) focuses on sensors imbedded into clothing for real-time, wireless transmission of physiologic information to a central server located within the home (Figure 11.3) (Tran, Cole, & Mendoza, 2002)."Smart" algorithms for processing and fusion of multiple wearable transducers may provide early, sensitive information regarding changes in physiologic status, simultaneous to evidence-based documentation of physiologic events that may be useful for long-term health care management. For example, a sensored vest worn by an elderly person with heart failure may serve to predict and avoid a catastrophic cardiac event via a combination of sensors that monitor heart rate variability, oxygen saturation levels, and alterations in blood pressure.

In addition to enabling frequent interaction with clinicians and real-time monitoring of health information, technology may play a third role, providing consumer biofeedback, in promoting health and disease prevention. Documentation and feedback of relevant information to elderly patients at home empower individuals for self-care. An example includes a technology-based approach to nutritional education for diabetes management. One scenario utilizes technology for monitoring nutritional intake by electronically recording consumption. Combined with physiologic recordings from commercially available glucometers, a software-guided nutrition plan may be implemented. Diabetics may be provided with real-time feedback regarding glucose abnormalities.

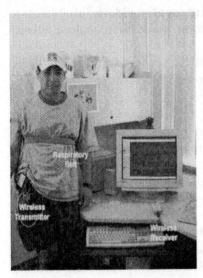 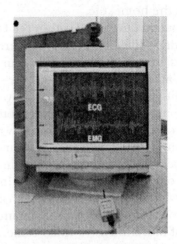

FIGURE 11.3   Wireless physiologic monitoring system with imbedded sensors for electrocardiogram (ECG), heart rate, electromyogram (EMG), and respiratory monitoring (wireless RF transmitter and receiver are highlighted).

This information may also be conveyed at appropriate instances to clinical personnel for interactive consultation with the diabetic consumer. Biermann, Dietrich, Rihl, and Standl (2002) have demonstrated savings in overall time and cost associated with management of insulin dependent diabetics using an integrated technological solution.

TECHNOLOGIES FOR PROMOTING INDEPENDENT LIVING

As noted elsewhere in this text, physical and cognitive disabilities, and the resultant loss of independence and increased safety concerns, present challenges to older adults wishing to age in place. Existing and emerging home automation technologies may, in part, provide means for improving independence and safety. Carefully placed sensors such as motion detectors, photo-detectors, and others coupled with automated devices for activating in-home lights can be used to improve ambient lighting conditions in the home environment, a major reason for falls by the elderly. Unobtrusive, low-cost sensors, switches, cameras, and other systems can be used to monitor and/or alert elderly inhabitants to various conditions, i.e., stove or iron left on, guests at front door, intruders in the home, etc.

A system developed within the HCTR Technology Center is designed to address these and other concerns. In contrast to most "smart" home efforts by other laboratories, our approach focuses on a consumer-affordable solution using off-the-shelf technologies capable of being retrofitted to existing living environments. A "consumer toolkit" of home automation and home monitoring devices has been developed that comprises motion sensors, switches, cameras, and appliance modules and is integrated with custom-design software for monitoring activities occurring within a home living environment (Cole & Tran, 2002). Low-cost sensors imbedded within the environment provide information, which can be correlated with activities of daily living. These sensors also continuously locate inhabitants' location within the living space in lieu of more intrusive video cameras. By constantly collecting information about activities being performed (i.e., ADLs, IADLs, etc.) and daily activity patterns, "smart" algorithms developed to detect changes in activity patterns may provide early indicators of changes in health status, onset of disability, or sensitive changes in cognitive abilities. Figure 11.4 shows an example of the set-up screen for the monitoring software along with graphical display of vital metrics being collected. This living laboratory environment has been implemented at the HCTR Technology Center. The software also is equipped with capabilities for two-way teleconsultation via Internet-based strategies between care providers and the user, as needed.

Further, the laboratory can be remotely observed over the Internet. Infrared sensors detecting motion within the environment activate several carefully situated cameras. Once activated, video images are automatically "pushed" to a Web server and can be accessed remotely over the Internet. The system can simultaneously monitor multiple cameras throughout the environment or can focus on fixed areas posing high safety risks (i.e., kitchen) to elderly persons. This system may be used for remote safety and security monitoring of a living environment by a caregiver or relatives.

An interactive living environment taking advantage of home automation, home monitoring, and home security, combined with Internet-based communications may promote successful aging in the elderly by enabling them to maintain control of their daily activities, ensuring safety and security, and by supporting independent living.

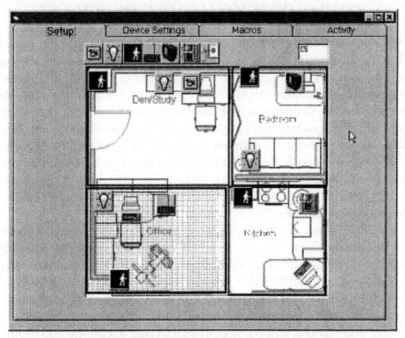

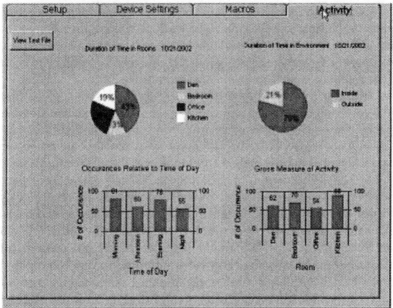

FIGURE 11.4 Unobtrusive monitoring software screen shots of (a) set-up screen and (b) output screen.

TECHNOLOGIES FOR LIFELONG ENGAGEMENT

A third major finding of the MacArthur Foundation studies on successful aging supported the need for *lifelong engagement*. Lifelong engagement was seen as instrumental in allaying onset of isolation, depression, and cognitive disabilities in elderly populations. Social and community supports for the maintenance of the elderly and those with chronic disabilities are important because advanced age and dysfunction (both physical and emotional) coincide with relative isolation among older people (Greenwald & Beery, 2001). For persons with disabilities, satisfaction with support systems was positively correlated to the adjustment to their disability, coping ability, psychosocial adaptation, and quality of life (McColl & Skinner, 1995).

As noted above, video telephony technology can be used to provide interactions between at-home patients and health care professionals. These systems may also be successfully used by family and friends for more personalized community-based support. Figure 11.5 shows three common configurations (i.e., set-top, desktop, and all-in-one) of POTS-based video telephony systems. Set-top systems (Figure 11.5a) are equipped with modem and camera, and connect to an external telephone and monitor for display. Desktop systems (Figure 11.5b) are equipped with modem, camera, and display, and connect to a standard telephone. All-in-one systems (Figure 11.5c) integrate all components (modem, camera, display, telephone) into one device. In general, purchase cost ranges from a few hundred dollars (a & b) to over a thousand dollars (c).

In addition, Internet-based interactive technologies such as discussion boards, chat rooms, instant messaging, and interactive video over Internet Protocol (IP), have been shown to alleviate isolation and depression in those with chronic conditions. Further investigation is required to evaluate the long-term benefits of these alternative mechanisms of social interaction. Technology-based interactive strategies for improving social interaction do not necessarily require high levels of ability or comfort with computers. Noncomputerized technologies such as WebTV™ (Microsoft Corp, Redmond, WA) and AOLTV™ (AOL Time Warner, New York, NY) enable Internet access and access to alternative communication venues via television monitors and set-top boxes.

Improved information and entertainment technologies also show promise for enhancing self-efficacy, supporting lifelong learning, and providing engaging activities for the elderly. Digital libraries provide widespread access to information and educational experiences for those

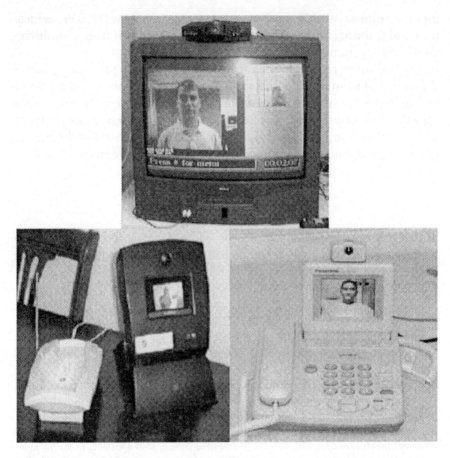

FIGURE 11.5 POTS-based video telephony systems (common types are (a) set-tops, (b) desktops, and (c) all-in-ones. Using low-cost sensors and home automation devices, a living space can easily be retrofitted to collect information about at-home users and their interactions with their environment for health monitoring purposes.

with Internet services in their homes. "Virtual reality" and immersive environments have the potential to provide interactive, engaging experiences for elderly individuals.

CONCLUSIONS

While technology has great potential to address the issues presented in this chapter, the key requirements to adoption of this technology include robust, reliable, and easy-to-use technology interfaces, education and training, and perhaps most important, buy-in from a multifaceted, heterogeneous group of end-users.

Despite these requirements, technology has great promise to fulfill the wishes of most older adults to successfully age in place and a host of technologies are now available to provide comprehensive services for a rapidly aging population . Combined, these technologies can promote independent living and successful aging by helping to avoid disease, to promote independence, and to enable lifelong engagement.

ACKNOWLEDGMENTS

Binh Q. Tran is Assistant Professor, HomeCare & Telerehabilitation Technology Center, Department of Biomedical Engineering, The Catholic University of America, Washington, D.C.

REFERENCES

American Heart Association (2002). *Heart disease and stroke statistics–2003*. Dallas, TX: Author

Biermann, E., Dietrich, W., Rihl, J., & Standl, E. (2002). Are there time and cost savings by using telemanagement for patients on intensified insulin therapy? *Computer Methods and Programs in Biomedicine, 69,* 137–146.

Buckley, K. M., Tran, B. Q., & Prandoni, C. (2001). *Nursing management and the acceptance/use of telehealth technologies by caregivers of stroke patients in the home setting.* Paper presented at the State-of-the-Sciences Conference on Telerehabilitation & Applications of Virtual Reality, Washington, D.C.

Cole, A., & Tran, B. Q. (2002). *Home automation to promote independent living in elderly populations.* Paper presented at the Joint Conference of the EMBS-BMES, Houston, Texas.

Fulmer, T., Feldman, P., Kim, T., Carty, B., Beers, M., Molina, M., & Putnam, M. (1999). An intervention study to enhance medication compliance in community-dwelling elderly individuals. *Journal of Gerontological Nursing, 25,* 6–14.

Gomez, E., Hernando, M., Garcia, A., Del Pozo, F., Cermeno, J., Corcoy, R., et al. (2002). Telemedicine as a tool for intensive management of diabetes: The DIABTel experience. *Computer Methods and Programs in Biomedicine, 69,* 163–177.

Greenwald, H., & Beery, W. (2001). Reducing isolation among inner-city elders: An outcome evaluation. *Journal of Health Promotion Practice, 2*(3), 233–241.

Guralnik, J., LaCroix, A., & Everett, D. (1989). *Aging in the eighties: The prevalence of comorbidity and its association with disability.* Hyattsville, MD: National Center for Health Statistics.

Kinsella, A. (1998). Telehealthcare in the management of CHF patients. *Caring,* 14–18.

Kinsella, A. (1999). *Improved care for diabetic populations: The need for telehealthcare and alternatives to conventional care services.* Paper presented at the Workshop on Home Care Technologies for the 21st Century, Washington D.C.

Kinsella, A. (2000a). Home telemedicine that "works." *Home Care Automation Report,* 7.

Kinsella, A. (2000b). Just Say "Hello"-Tele-Interventions for Diabetes Care. *Home Care Automation Report,* 2–3.

McColl, M., & Skinner, H. (1995). Assessing inter- and intrapersonal resources: Social support and coping among adults with a disability. *Disability Rehab,* 17(1), 24–34.

The Robert Wood Johnson Foundation (1998). *Chronic care in America: A 21st century challenge.* Princeton, NJ: Author.

Rowe, J. W., & Kahn, R. L. (1998). *Successful aging.* New York: Pantheon Books.

Shah, N. B., Der, E., Ruggerio, C., Heindenreich, P. A., & Massie, B. M. (1998). Prevention of hospitalizations for heart failure with an interactive home monitoring program. *American Heart Journal, 135,* 373–378.

Tran, B., Cole, A., & Mendoza, G. (2002). *Wireless technologies: Biomedical applications and implementations in the home.* Paper presented at the Sarnoff Symposium (IEEE), Advances in Wired and Wireless Communications, Ewing, New Jersey.

Tran, B. Q., Buckley, K. M., & Prandoni, C. M. (2002). Selection and use of telehealth technology in support of homebound caregivers of stroke patients. *Caring, 21*(3), 16–21.

Tran, B. Q., Kinsella, A., Winters, J., Thiel, L., Prandoni, C., & Hughes, E. (1999). *Utility of mass-market technologies to enable care provided by laypersons in the home environment.* Paper presented at the First Joint Meeting of Biomedical Engineering Society & Engineering in Medicine and Biology Society.

Tran, B. Q., Krainak, D. M., Lauderdale, D. E., & Winters, J. M. (2002). Video telephony in tele-health care: Accessible and emerging technologies. In C. R. J. Winters, R. Simpson, & G. Vanderheiden (Eds.), *Emerging and accessible telecommunications, information, and health care technologies-engineering challenges in enabling universal access.* Arlington, VA: RESNA Press.

U.S. Census Bureau (1997). *American with disabilities, 1994–95.* Available at www.census.gov/main.cprs.html

U.S. Census Bureau (2001). Statistics.

U.S. Department of Health & Human Services (2000). *Healthy People 2010.* Paper presented at the Partnerships for Health in the New Millennium Conference, Washington, D.C.

Section D

Models, Prototypes, and
Specific Applications
of Gerotechnology

12

Technology and the Culture of Change: Application of Aviation Human Factors Research to Health Care Systems

K. Victor Ujimoto

The application of technology to enhance the well-being of the elderly poses a fundamental challenge, stemming in most instances from the fact that technological devices are often introduced as a substitute for human resources, mainly for economic reasons. The decision to utilize technology is also often made without an understanding of the social and cultural characteristics of the intended users. The key question that arises is whether or not the application of technology in its various forms actually enhances the well-being of the elderly.

In order to better understand the relationship between the application of technology and its impact on the well-being of the elderly, it is first necessary to understand more precisely the concept of technology-practice. For baby boomers raised in the postindustrial era, the meaning of technology did not extend beyond its technical or physical meanings, for example, tools, machines, computers, etc. In contrast, for those who examined the social relations, social control, and the social shaping of technology, for example, Pacey (1984), and MacKenzie and Wajcman, (1999), the focus was primarily on the administrative, management, or organizational aspects of the application of technology. Therefore, in the application of technology, in our case for the well-being of the elderly, the key components of technology-practice as articulated by Pacey will be used to frame our discussion in this chapter.

It should be noted that our examination of these key components as an integrative whole forces us to a new style of "systemic thinking" through which a person "perceives reciprocity, connections, and inter-dependencies" (Theobald, 1972, p. 10). Although systemic thinking was advanced in the early 1960s, it is still an approach that is often ignored by important decision makers today in everyday life. A continuing challenge is to create a new awareness of the relationship between technology and its application to enhance the well-being of the elderly.

THE MEANING OF TECHNOLOGY

As Pacey (1984) has stated, there is a wide range of social and cultural content in technology-practice. Of particular interest in our examination of technology and cultural change are the goals, personal values, beliefs, and ethics of both the caregivers and medical staff in administering to the needs and well-being of the elderly. Pacey quotes J. K. Galbraith's definition of technology as "the systematic application of scientific or other organized knowledge to practical tasks."

Pacey expands on Galbraith's definition to include "liveware" as well as hardware, to define technology-practice as "the application of scientific and other knowledge to practical tasks by ordered systems that involve people and organizations, living things and machines." Recently, the inclusion and integration of "liveware," organizations, and machines has advanced considerably in the aviation flight safety and error management literature. A brief overview of this literature will illustrate the importance of understanding the culture of a group or an organization in relation to technology. Several of the concepts noted here can also be applied to the introduction of technology to enhance the safety and well-being of the elderly.

TECHNOLOGY AND HUMAN FACTORS

The study of technology's relationship to people can be captured in the field of human factors and ergonomics (Hawkins, 1993; Fisk & Rogers, 1997; and Rogers, 1997). One of the earliest studies of the relationship between technology and human performance was the integrative model advanced by Edwards (Hawkins, 1993). This model, based on the SHEL concept, examined the relationship between software, hardware, environment, and liveware. The central component or hub of the model is the person or liveware to which we had referred earlier. Hawkins notes that it is essential to understand the characteristics of this central component as they relate to the other components of the socio-technical system.

A crucial characteristic of a person or liveware is the person's physical dimensions. There must be an appropriate fit between the person and his or her environment (Kroemer, 1997). In the case of the elderly, the individual's physical dimensions may vary according to age, ethnicity, and sex. Yet, very often "one size fits all" technical devices seem to be the norm. Thus, the application of human factors may have future payoffs. Other aspects of human factors or liveware considerations are the nutritional, physiological, and psychological aspects of well-being that can be influenced or modified by various technological devices.

Hawkins notes variability in information processing capabilities across individuals as another human factor or liveware issue. As noted in earlier chapters, information processing ability generally declines with age, so we are challenged to carefully judge individuals' information processing abilities in order not to compromise safety and well-being. When individuals can no longer monitor their own technological assistive devices, caregivers must take on this responsibility. As Hawkins suggests, the monitoring instrument or warning system design must consider the capabilities and limitations of the human information processing system. This is particularly important when there are sensory and cognitive deficiencies as one ages (Craik, 1977; Hultsch & Dixon, 1990; Smith, 1996). Thus, redundancy mechanisms should be incorporated into the socio-technical system to assist the elderly to cope with memory losses, for example, devices to remind them to take medicine, about doctor's appointments, etc., as well as other relevant health information such as warnings not to mix medications.

Hardware comprises the second key component of the SHEL model. The liveware-hardware fit or interface must be flexible enough to adjust to the various sensory, motor, and cognitive characteristics of the person. If the fit is not perfect, injury may occur that results in pain or even permanent disability. Hawkins (1993) has also noted that the individual's information processing capabilities must be considered when evaluating a liveware-hardware interface. Several control devices for making hardware adjustments are based on the individual's ability to process necessary information prior to adjusting hardware controls.

An example of incorrect information resulting in a fatal medical error occurred at the Duke University Medical Center on February 7, 2003. A mismatched blood-type in a heart and lung transplant operation resulted in the death of 17-year-old Jessica Santillan. A second operation was scheduled, but it was too late and Jessica died. Here, the liveware-hardware fit was imperfect because liveware characteristics such as blood type and immune system status were not accurately checked and rechecked (Vergano, 2003). This is part of the overall systems procedures, which is in the realm of software.

The liveware-software interface is the second interface we will consider. The software encompasses those aspects of the socio-technical system such as computer programs, systems procedures, checklists, and other subprograms built into the overall socio-technical system. Again, systems operators must understand integrative aspects of the software components. As illustrated in our tragic example above, inadequate understanding of essential components and functions may result in serious accidents.

Procedures employed in any systems operations are only as effective as the training of system operators and it is critically important for operators to follow established functions and associated checklists in order to reduce errors. This can only be achieved through a positive institutional or organizational culture that instills in each employee a sense of responsibility for safety. This aspect of organizational culture will be discussed in greater detail later in this chapter.

The third interface consideration is between liveware and the environment. Environment refers both to the institutional environment of the elderly and the work environment of the caregivers and medical staff. Important considerations of the environments include noise levels, temperature variations, air quality, and lighting intensity. With much existing technology the environment can be adjusted to meet human requirements. For example, air conditioning systems can be installed to control for both temperature and humidity. Economic considerations rather than available technology are often the decisive factor when selecting a technology.

The final interface consideration is the liveware to liveware interface. Here, the elder's interaction with staff will depend on factors such as personality, interests, and socio-economic status. The interaction patterns are not limited to client-staff relations but include interaction among staff and administration of different levels. Here again, institutional or organizational culture becomes important because cooperation or teamwork among systems personnel is important for the smooth functioning of the overall socio-technical system. A lack of teamwork can result in safety violations or systems breakdown.

TECHNOLOGY, CULTURE, AND SYSTEM ERRORS

The importance of understanding the relationship between technology, culture, and human behavior has been noted earlier. One obvious reason for this is to prevent errors, incidents, and accidents from occurring in any socio-technical system. A single isolated error may not result in any serious outcome; however, an accumulating series of errors may combine to create organizational accidents leading to injury or death. Human performance of critical tasks can be facilitated by the introduction of technology; however, the operators of socio-technical systems must be vigilant, particularly in a healthcare system where mistakes can be deadly.

Organizational accidents can occur in any modern socio-technical system and often have multiple causes. Accidents do not generally occur at a single level but are spread throughout the organization. Unfortunately, if a serious accident does not occur for a long time, a steady erosion of protection often results (Reason, 1997). It is therefore necessary to establish effective protection or defenses to prevent accidents. Such protections should include understanding and awareness of local hazards, clear guidance on how to operate safely, alarms and warnings of imminent danger, systems restored to a safe state in an off-normal situation, safety barriers interposed between hazards and potential losses, containment and elimination of hazards should they escape this barrier, and provision for escape and rescue should hazard containment fail.

Thus, as an integral part of the liveware-software interface, the procedural functions are distinctly separate from the technological aspects of the hardware. Today's use of computers and other automated monitoring devices in many institutional settings very often neglects the protective and safety considerations. Reason has outlined a functional hierarchy of defenses that act as successive or multiple layers of protection. However, under certain conditions, these successive layers themselves will be subject to unsafe conditions or situations.

Reason's "Swiss cheese" model of defenses which can be adapted to the health care system, depicts multiple layers of necessary protection. Each slice of the cheese represents the various sectors or departments within institutions such as hospitals or long term care facilities. Each sector or department providing direct or indirect patient care is a potential source for some mistake or error. These are represented metaphorically by the holes in the Swiss cheese, symbolizing the weaknesses in the organization that can shift around within a sector or department depending on such factors as workloads, staff changes, shift work schedules, and lack of training, communications, or adherence to established procedures.

Reason's model differentiates "holes" by considering the important distinction between "active failures" and "latent conditions" inherent in any socio-technical system. "Unsafe acts are likely to have a direct impact on the safety of the system, and because of the immediacy of their adverse effects, these acts are termed active failures" (p. 10). Here again, we are referring to the human factors or liveware considerations that contribute to the breakdown in the safe operation of the socio-technical system. Human decisions and actions based on lapses in memory, poor judgment, and violations in procedures are prime examples of active failures.

In contrast to active failures, Reason (1997) notes, "latent conditions are to technological organizations what resident pathogens are to the human body. Like pathogens, latent conditions—such as poor design, gaps in supervision, undetected manufacturing defects or maintenance failures, unworkable procedures, clumsy automation, shortfalls in training, and inadequate tools and equipment—may exist for many years before they combine with local circumstances and active failures to penetrate the system's many layers of defenses" (p. 10). In this distinction between active failures and latent conditions, two important organizational factors should be noted: (a) the time factor between the active failure(s) and the adverse impact, and (b) the specific location within the organization where the human factors flaws originate. To illustrate these two points, Reason (1997) notes that "active failures are committed by those humans at the human-system interface, and they usually have immediate and short-lived effects" (p. 11). These contrast with latent conditions such as original design flaws or undetected manufacturing defects, which can be dormant for years before system defenses are breached and an accident occurs. These latent conditions can be blamed on the earlier decision makers at the top of the organizational hierarchy. In order to examine why active failures and latent conditions continue to exist in contemporary socio-technical systems and organizations, we will next examine the relationship between technology, corporate or institutional culture, and systems safety.

SOCIO-TECHNICAL SYSTEMS, ORGANIZATIONAL CULTURE, AND SYSTEM SAFETY

In most studies of catastrophic system failures, the conclusion reached was that an accumulation of failures and errors scattered throughout the socio-technical system, either during manufacture or at some other decision-making level of an organization, were responsible for the accident (Stewart, 1994; Vaughan, 1996). Most failures or violations in system procedure appears to be associated with the lack of a strong institutional or organizational culture.

Westrum and Adamski (1999) present another way to consider the relationship between the socio-technical system, the liveware discussed in the SHEL model, and the linkage to Reason's notion of active and latent failures. "Around every complex operation there is a human envelope that develops, operates, maintains, interfaces, and evaluates the functioning of the sociotechnical system" (p. 69).

In Westrum and Adamski's model, members of the human envelope are held together by the organization's culture. They define this organizational culture as "an ensemble of patterns of thought, feeling, and behavior that guide the action of the organization's members" (p. 81). Although individuals may act alone, it is through their interaction with others that organizational cultural patterns develop based on a common set of beliefs, values, and norms. Trice and Beyer (1993) note this as the collective characteristic of culture and they assert that "belonging to a culture involves believing what others believe and doing as they do—at least part of the time" (p. 5). Other important characteristics of culture noted by Trice and Beyer are "the emotional, historical, symbolic, dynamic, and inherently fuzzy" aspects.

In examining the relationship between socio-technical systems and organizational culture, the emotional characteristics of culture are particularly significant because of what people believe and cherish. The introduction of technology that requires social change may very well result in considerable resistance to change in fundamental behavior because of established ideologies and practices. "People's allegiances to their ideologies and cultural forms thus spring more from their emotional needs than from national considerations" (Trice & Beyer, 1999, p. 6).

The development of emotional culture often results from people sharing common histories or experiences. If the introduction of technology into an organization replaces human beings, there will be no opportunity for people to interact with others and they merely become a part of an emotionless environment. An example is the numerically programmed medication dispenser that moves along hospital corridors to deliver prescribed drugs. The patient merely steps outside his or her room around the prescribed time to pick up his or her medicine. There will be limited opportunity to interact with traditional nurses or other caregivers, thus preventing a meaningful exchange of daily greetings and conversation.

An important aspect of both the emotional and historical dimensions of culture for the well-being of elders is to remember their need to spend time together and to interact with staff members if a strong organizational culture is to be developed and strengthened. This is unlikely to occur if there are more temporary or short-term contract personnel employed than there are regular staff members. Although it may be economically advantageous to employ part-time staff or to introduce technological devices for repetitive or routine tasks, the major disadvantage will be the absence of a strong organizational culture that can produce new ideas or innovations to make gradual, continuous improvements to the socio-technical system.

The significance of the symbolic aspects of culture has been noted by Trice and Beyer (1993) who write, "to say that cultures are symbolic is to emphasize the expressive, rather than the technical and practical side of human behavior" (p. 6). In our multicultural society, symbolism plays an important role in facilitating cross-cultural communication and understanding. Individuals must be encouraged to manifest their cultural expressions freely instead of being restricted or limited by technological determinism. The opportunities for cultural expression enhance and facilitate the development of the dynamic aspects of culture.

In our examination of the relationship between socio-technical systems and organizational culture, there are several reasons why one must fully understand the dynamic nature of culture across generations. Trice and Beyer (1993) provide five explanations of why cultures continually change. First, because communication is seldom perfect, the transfer of knowledge from one generation to the next is also imperfect and successive generations will interpret their past culture in different ways. Second, individuals have considerable discretion to create their own patterns of behavior. Trice and Beyer (1993) note that "the degree of individualism varies across societies over time but is probably always sufficient to produce some degree of innovativeness and creativity in responding to life's problems and challenges" (p. 7). Third, cultures change because so much of the traditional elements of a culture are taken for granted and thus not assessed in terms of their meanings to specific contemporary events or issues. Fourth, the emphasis on the symbolic aspects of communication results in imprecise interpretations. Finally, new groups, new technologies, and concomitant new practices result in new organizational environments that produce a fluid, dynamic, organizational culture.

The final characteristic of culture noted by Trice and Beyer (1993) is the "inherently fuzzy" aspect of contemporary cultures. These "incorporate contradictions, ambiguities, paradoxes, and just plain confusion most often manifested in modern organizations operating in uncertain and confusing environments" (p. 7). The resulting fuzziness stems from several sources such as the imperfect transmission of previous cultural values, shared rules, and norms, and the influence of new subcultural groups that emerge in an organization as a result of the introduction of new technologies and organizational practices.

An understanding of the various characteristics of culture will enable us to appreciate the model advanced by Westrum and Adamski (1999) to study the relationship between technology, organizational culture, and system safety. The ultimate goal is the safe operation of the sociotechnical system. In order to minimize the exposure of the elderly to dangerous situations that may be associated with various day to day activities and practices in a hospital or in a nursing home environment, we will next briefly discuss those factors of organizational culture that most specifically concern system safety. Westrum and Adamski identify three types of organizational cultures—pathological, bureaucratic, and generative. The flow of information varies in each type and affects the efficiency, productivity, and safety of that organization.

In pathological organizations the anomalies, system errors, or mistakes are not transmitted beyond the immediate confines of the work or operational environment. The suppression of any adverse situation or "latent pathogens" does not eradicate the problem but is hidden from view until a major disaster is experienced. As Westrum and Adamski (1999) note, "the suppression or encapsulation of the problem does not make the problem go away, just the message about it. Such organizations constantly generate 'latent pathogens,' since internal political forces act without concern for integrity" (p. 84). This situation usually remains undetected unless the organizational and political cultures embrace rather than punish "whistle-blowers." Many hospitals and nursing homes in Canada and the U.S. tend to follow the pathological organizational culture and structure.

Bureaucratic organizations rely on highly complex socio-technical fixes. These organizations "tend to be good at routine or predictable problems. They do not actively create pathogens at the rate of pathological organizations, but they are not very good at spotting or fixing them" (Westrum and Adamski, 1999, p. 84). Staff in these organizations show a tendency to take a very narrow or "linear thinking" approach and do not consider issues that occur beyond the assigned area of their job description or responsibility. An example of such a bureaucratic organization is one where each department has its own computer operating system that cannot communicate with systems in other departments. Thus, issues arising in one department are not readily shared across the whole organization. Consequently, an organizational culture that reinforces the "why bother?" mentality sets in and eventually becomes part of the latent failure.

Generative organizations encourage information sharing through good communications. Westrum and Adamski note that "the generative organization possesses a high degree of integrity, a human envelope in depth that protects the socio-technical system. When the system occasionally generates a latent pathogen, the problem is likely to be quickly spotted and fixed" (p. 85). The generative organization is perhaps best illustrated by the many aviation organizations that have a nearly perfect safety record (Gittell, 2003). In the airline industry, the main focus is on the management of system safety and this can only be accomplished effectively through an organizational culture that successfully integrates operational, technical, and human resources. This integrative approach to the study of system safety developed with the very first examination of the nontechnical aspects of aviation accidents after the tragic crash of the Lockheed L-1011 in Florida in 1972. In this accident, the National Transportation Safety Board (NTSB) of the United States attributed the main cause of the accident to "the failure of the crew to monitor the flight instruments during the final four minutes of flight, and to detect an unexpected descent soon enough to prevent impact with the ground" (Lauber, 1993, p. xv).

Since then, research has accelerated on flight crew performance and how human factors issues affected their operations (Ujimoto, 2002). The main research thrust commenced in the mid 1970s at the NASA Ames Research Center. In 1979 a workshop entitled "Resource Management on the Flight Deck" was held (Cooper, White, & Lauber, 1980) and several human factors issues were identified such as human error, poor interpersonal communication, failure to set priorities in decision making, loss in situation awareness, and inadequate leadership.

The original expansion of cockpit resource management (CRM) to crew resource management (CRM) occurred with the recognition that increased flight safety and efficiency required a cooperative or "team effort" between the flight deck and flight attendants. Orlady and Orlady (1999) have noted that in the early days of aviation, human characteristics such as individualism and independence were viewed as desirable pilot characteristics; however, with the introduction of the copilot and technological advancements in the cockpit, this view changed. This worthwhile objective adhered to the original definition of CRM provided by Lauber (1984) as "the effective utilization of all available resources—hardware, software, and liveware—to achieve safe, efficient flight operations" (p. 20).

Several important aspects should be noted in Lauber's definition. First, the meaning of "effective utilization" has been interpreted in various ways. In western societies, where rugged individualism and independence predominate, much greater emphasis appears to be placed on the economic aspects of flight operations rather than on flight safety through teamwork. Second, the scope of "resources" today must be extended beyond the flight crew environment, and the overall aviation or air transport system must be considered. This argument will become more obvious when we analyze the various processes and causes of errors that result in aviation accidents and incidents. Third, flight operations as an organizational system comprises many subsystems and the role of each subsystem must be understood and appreciated as an important component of the overall air transport system.

Crew resource management as an overarching principle for flight safety required several decades of nourishment before it gained recognition throughout the aviation industry. However, there are still critics of CRM because accidents continue to occur because of human errors. Helmreich (2000) notes that "critics of CRM fail to recognize two vital points: (a) that humans are inherently limited in their capabilities, making error inevitable; and (b) that complex systems such as aviation will necessarily experience failures" (p. ix). Similarly, in health care settings, human errors can occur when highly complex technological systems are introduced. Recognizing the limitations of human capabilities and compensating for them through a more effective understanding of human factors can reduce errors. These factors include better training and the development of a strong organizational culture.

SUMMARY AND CONCLUSION

This chapter has provided an overview of the diverse social and cultural contexts of technology-practice. It was noted that the application of technology to enhance the well-being of the elderly must be from a systems perspective that integrates the software, hardware, and environment with liveware. Literature addressing the relationship between technology, organizational culture, and aging is growing gradually; however, there is still not enough emphasis on interdisciplinary systems approaches. This chapter's brief overview of the progress made in aviation human factors and safety research seeks to encourage better collaboration among disciplines with regard to future technology, human factors, and research on aging. This will undoubtedly become quite urgent in future years as assistive technology is continually introduced into medical care systems.

The introduction of technology to address broad-based health care issues must stem from a firm understanding of both technology and organizational culture. Without this understanding, especially from a systems or teamwork perspective, compromises may occur in the health care system that will result in an increase in technology-generated iatrogenic and nosocomial morbidity and mortality. The success of aviation human factors and CRM research is now gaining attention in the medical profession. Helmreich and Merritt (1998) note the importance of interpersonal collaboration, communication, and coordination in the working environment for both commercial airline pilots and medical operating room teams. But this emphasis on safety still lags in the medical profession. For example, the U.S. Federal Aviation Administration (FAA) and the National Aeronautics and Space Administration (NASA) established the Aviation Safety Reporting System (ASRS), a nonpunitive incident reporting system in 1975. Orlady and Orlady (1999) report that pilots, flight attendants, mechanics, technicians, and other airline personnel file nearly 3000 anonymous reports each month. If the medical and health care professionals adopted a similar anonymous reporting system, for example a Medical Safety Reporting System (MSRS), perhaps there would be far fewer medical errors.

This example points to some improvements that can be obtained by a shared interactive information technology system that disseminates interdisciplinary information on medical and health care safety issues. Modern information technology can greatly facilitate and enhance our interdisciplinary sharing of knowledge; and medical terminology can enhance all aspects of treatment and care. However, the introduction of technology must be made with a firm commitment to the understanding of the organizational culture of the institutional environment.

ACKNOWLEDGMENTS

K. Victor Ujimoto is affiliated with the Commercial Aviation Program, University of Western Ontario, London, Ontario, Canada.

REFERENCES

Craik, F. I. M. (1977). Age differences in human memory. In J. E. Birren & K. W. Schaie (Eds.), *Handbook of the psychology of aging*. New York: Van Nostrand Reinhold.

Cooper, G. E., White, M. D., & Lauber, J. K. (1980). *Resource management on the flight deck: Proceedings of a NASA/industry workshop*. Moffett Field, CA: NASA Ames Research Center.

Fisk, A. D., & Rogers, W. A. (1997). *Handbook of human factors and the older adult*. New York: Academic Press.

Gittell, J. H. (2003). *The Southwest airliner way*. New York: McGraw-Hill.

Hawkins, F. H. (1993). *Human factors in flight*. Aldershot, England: Ashgate Publishing.

Helmreich, R. L. (2000). *Forward: Human factors and aerospace safety, 1*(1), p. ix.

Helmreich, R. L., & Merritt, A. C. (1998). *Culture at work in aviation and medicine*. Aldershot, England: Ashgate.

Hultsch, D. F., & Dixon, R. A. (1990). Learning and memory in aging. In J. E. Birren & K. W. Schaie (Eds.), *Handbook of the psychology of aging*. New York: Academic Press.

Kroemer, K. H. E. (1997). Anthropometry and biomechanics. In A. D. Fisk & W. A. Rogers (Eds.), *Handbook of human factors and the older adult*. New York: Academic Press.

Lauber, J. K. (1984). Resource management in the cockpit. *Airline Pilot, 5*, 20–23.

Lauber, J. K. (1993). Foreword. In E. L. Wiener, B. G. Kanki, & R. L. Helmreich (Eds.), *Cockpit resource management*. New York: Academic Press.

MacKenzie, D., & Wajcman, J. (1999). *The social shaping of technology*. Buckingham, UK: Open University Press.

Orlady, H. W., & Orlady, L. M. (1999). *Human factors in multi-crew flight operations*. Aldershot, England: Ashgate.

Pacey, A. (1984). *The culture of technology*. Cambridge, MA: The MIT Press.

Reason, J. (1997). *Managing the risks of organizational accidents*. Brookfield, Vermont: Ashgate.

Rogers, W. A. (1997). Individual differences, aging, and human factors: An overview. In A. D. Fisk & W. A. Rogers (Eds.), *Handbook of human factors and the older adult*. New York: Academic Press.

Smith, A. D. (1996). Memory. In J. E. Birren & K. W. Schaie (Eds.), *Handbook of the psychology of aging*. New York: Academic Press.

Stewart, S. (1994). *Air disasters: Dialogue from the black box*. Enderby, Australia: Bookmark Limited.

Theobald, R. (1972). *Habit and habitat*. Englewood Cliffs, NJ: Prentice-Hall.

Trice, H. M., & Beyer, J M. (1993). *The cultures of work organizations*. Englewood Cliffs, NJ: Prentice-Hall.

Ujimoto, K. V. (2002). Human factors in air transport operations: From flight crew to corporate resource management. In T. Oum (Ed.), *Proceedings of the 6th air transport research society conference (ATRS)*. Seattle: Boeing Training Center.

Vaughn, D. (1996). *The Challenger launch decision: Risky technology, culture, and deviance at NASA*. Chicago: University of Chicago Press.

Vergano, D. (2003). Near-fatal transplant mistake being investigated. *USA Today*, February 21, p. 2A.

Westrum, R., & Adamski, A. J. (1999). Organizational Factors Associated With Safety and Mission Success in Aviation Environments. In D. J. Garland, J. A. Wise, & V. D. Hopkin (Eds.), *Handbook of aviation human factors*. Mahwah, NJ: Lawrence Erlbaum Associates.

13

Driving Simulation
and Older Adults

George W. Rebok and Penelope M. Keyl

Doctor, we are concerned that my 82-year-old father is no longer safe to drive even though he recently passed a driving evaluation at the Department of Motor Vehicles. He is only driving locally, but has gotten lost several times and has had several near-miss road situations. We've advised him that he is unsafe and is going to hurt himself, his wife, and other people. Although we've offered to drive him anywhere he needs to go, he insists that he is a safe driver and that he has no intention of quitting. We don't want him to cause an accident, but we are not sure what to do next.

The population of older people in the United States is growing dramatically (U.S. Bureau of the Census, 2003), and a concomitant increase in the prevalence of dementia is expected. Thus, as the above vignette illustrates, the issue of safety, particularly driver safety, in older people is becoming a growing public health concern, and one for which interventions are being sought (Carr & Wang, 2003). According to the National Highway Traffic Safety Administration (NHTSA), although older drivers have the lowest crash rate per licensed driver of all (driving) age groups (NHTSA, 2001a), they also have higher crash rates per vehicle mile driven and higher fatality rates from crashes (NHTSA, 2001b), due in part to their greater susceptibility to physical injury (Li, Braver, & Chen, 2003). In fact, based on estimated annual travel, the fatality rate for drivers age 85 years and older is nine times higher than for drivers 25–69 years old (NHTSA, 2001b). Increased crash rates in elderly drivers have been attributed to age-related declines in visual search, selective and divided attention, and complex reaction time (Ball & Rebok, 1994; Ball, Owsley, Sloane, Roenker, & Bruni, 1993; Owsley, Ball, Sloane, Roenker, & Bruni, 1991; Stutts, Stewart, & Martell, 1998), as well as the presence of medical diseases (Wallace, 1997).

As also illustrated by the introductory vignette, the responsibility for determining the driving fitness of older adults is increasingly falling upon the health care profession. Although medical professionals need to be equipped with objective methods to evaluate fitness to drive (Carr & Rebok, 2000; Freund, Gravenstein, Ferris, & Shaheen, 2002), they often do so with minimal objective data on which to base a decision. The ultimate decision as to whether a patient should continue to drive is made by the local licensing authority, but the physician can influence this process. Physicians also have an ethical responsibility to notify the appropriate authorities when the patient poses a threat to others (Kakaiya, Tisovec, & Fulkerson, 2000).

During the past decade driving simulation has begun to play an increasingly important role in assessing driving fitness and retraining driving skills in older drivers. This chapter will review the uses and validity of driving simulation technology with the elderly, focusing on the following issues: 1) review and critical evaluation of the existing research on driving simulation in the elderly; 2) comparison of the feasibility and validity of driving simulation approaches to other methods for assessing driving ability (e.g., on-road driving, neuropsychological assessment); 3) use of driving simulators for retraining or rehabilitating elderly drivers who present driving problems; and 4) combining simulator technology with functional magnetic resonance imaging (fMRI) and other neuroimaging technologies to study underlying neural mechanisms.

SIMULATION STUDIES WITH OLDER DRIVERS

Driving simulation has occupied an important place in automobile human factors research for more than two decades. Simulator research topics include driver interaction with suspension and steering systems (Blana & Golias, 2002; Hildreth, Beusmans, Boer, & Royden, 2000), driver workload (Hicks & Wierwille, 1979; Jerome, Ganey, Mouloua, & Hancock, 2002; Verwey, 2000), and the effects of alcohol and drugs on driver performance (Quillian, Cox, Kovatchev, & Phillips, 1999; Gawron & Ranney, 1988; McGinty, Shih, Garrett, Calhoun, & Pearlson, 2001). Recently, driving simulation has been extended to the study of driving behaviors of healthy older drivers and those with physical and cognitive impairments. Because simulators allow investigators to examine driving behaviors and conditions that would be too hazardous for on-road assessment, they have become increasingly popular in automotive human factors research with the elderly (Alexander, Barham, & Black, 2002; Hakamies-Blomqvist, Ostlund, & Hneroksson, 2000; Staplin, 1995). Advances in computers, image processing, and display and sensor technologies in the last decade have also facilitated the development of simulation systems that are more interactive and that more closely mirror real-world driving conditions at reasonable cost, which has led to increased use in both public and private sectors (Emery, Robin, Knipling, Finn, & Fleger, 1999; Gruening, Bernard, Clover, & Hoffmeister, 1998; Lee & Mollenhauer, 2002; Tornros, 1998; Weir & Clark 1996).

Several studies have examined the relationship between age-related perceptual and cognitive changes and driving simulator performance. Some have been conducted among participants with no known neurocognitive impairments, whereas others have been conducted among patients with physical and/or cognitive impairments resulting from conditions such as Alzheimer's disease and stroke. The major objective of this research has been to predict who is likely to be an unsafe driver. Although it is not always feasible for everyone to have an expensive, high-performance driving simulator to assess driving abilities, it is feasible to use lower-tech, easily administered neuropsychogical procedures that correlate highly with simulation data and real-life crash data (Keyl, Rebok, & Gallo, 1997).

SIMULATION STUDIES WITH HEALTHY OLDER ADULTS

Several simulation studies with healthy older adults have compared performance on a simulator with a measure of visual processing speed for increasingly more difficult attention tasks called the "useful field of view" (UFOV®). Much of the interest in the notion of useful field of view in general and the computer-based UFOV® measure in particular stems from its ability to predict crashes with high sensitivity and specificity, especially among older adults (Ball, Wadley, & Edwards, 2002). For example, Roenker, Cissell, and Ball conducted a study (cited in Ball & Owsley, 2000) examining driving simulator performance in relation to the UFOV®. Older individuals with intact visual acuity and contrast sensitivity were assessed in a Doron Model L-225 driving simulator. The Doron simulator is a fixed-base, noninteractive system consisting of a single driving station with a steering wheel and a typical instrument panel.

Results of this study identified a significant relationship between UFOV® and simple reaction time to brake lights as well as choice reaction time to varying traffic signs. Individuals with greater UFOV® impairment demonstrated slower choice response times in the driving simulator. In another study Chaparro, Groff, Tabor, Sifrit, and Gugerty (1999) examined the relationship between UFOV® and a test of situational awareness in driving (DriveSim). DriveSim is administered on a desktop personal computer and shows a three-dimensional scene representing the view from inside a car, including the roadway, vehicles ahead, and rearview, right, and left sideview mirrors. Participants ranging in age from 18 to 82 were administered a battery of tests including the UFOV® and instructed to monitor the number and location of all vehicles in the scene and to avoid collisions. Performance on UFOV® subtests 2 and 3 (divided and selective attention) was significantly correlated with DriveSim accident involvement, ability to recognize and react to a threat car, and the average proportion of cars recalled.

Cox, Taylor, and Kovatchev (1999) studied 38 older people who three years previously had participated in a driving simulation study using an Atari driving simulator. The Atari simulator has three 25-inch computer screens that wrap around the driver providing a 165-degree visual field, and a programmed rearview mirror depicting rear traffic. Twenty of the 38 drivers had scored above the 90th percentile (low risk), and 18 had scored below the 10th percentile (high risk) on the driving simulator test. Although both high- and low-risk drivers reported driving a similar number of miles per week, the high-risk drivers reported 47 crashes per 1,000,000 miles driven whereas the low-risk drivers reported six crashes per 1,000,000 miles, a significant difference that persisted when controlling for age.

SIMULATION STUDIES WITH ALZHEIMER'S PATIENTS

Several recent studies have used simulators to determine driving fitness in patients with Alzheimer's disease. For example, Rizzo, Reinach, McGhee, and Dawson (1997) examined driving simulator performance in 21 older adults with Alzheimer's disease and 18 age-matched controls without dementia. Participants "drove" on a simulated rural two-lane highway in the Iowa Driving Simulator, SIREN (Simulator for Interdisciplinary Research in Ergonomics and Neuroscience). The SIREN is a four-channel, 150 degree forward view and 50 degree rear view high-fidelity simulator that provides a dynamic driving scenario in which "crashes" are recorded. Six (29%) of 21 participants with Alzheimer's experienced crashes vs. none of the 18 control participants. Among 15 participants with total UFOV® impairment of 50% or greater, 6 had at least one crash, while none of the control participants with total UFOV® loss less than 50% had any crashes. Correlations between UFOV® impairment and simulator crashes were of a magnitude similar to that reported by Ball, Owsley, Sloane, Roenker, and Bruni (1993) with state-recorded crashes.

In an earlier series of studies on simulated driving in Alzheimer's disease, Rebok and colleagues (Rebok, Bylsma, & Keyl, 1990; Bylsma, 1997; Bylsma, Rebok, & Keyl, 1992; Rebok, Keyl, Bylsma, Blaustein, & Tune, 1994) examined driving performance in relation to a broad battery of cognitive function tests. Rebok, Keyl, Bylsma, Blaustein and Tune (1994) reported that Alzheimer's patients' performance on two cognitive tests, the Mini-Mental State Examination (MMSE) and a test of category fluency, correlated significantly with aspects of their performance on a quasi-simulation of driving using the Driving Advisement System (DAS)(Gianutsos, 1992). In a larger, follow-up study, 42 patients with Alzheimer's and 81 healthy elderly control subjects participated in an 18-month longitudinal study to evaluate automobile driving skills using the Doron driving simulator. First visit test results on several measures of neuropsychological function (i.e., Trails A, Motor-Free Visual Perception Test, Visual Reproduction, mean reaction time in 2- and 4-choice reaction time tests) were significantly associated with driving simulator performance for both the Alzheimer's patients and controls (Rebok, Bylsma, & Keyl, 1990; Bylsma, Rebok, & Keyl, 1992). In a longitudinal analysis of subjects with three visits, Rebok, Keyl, Bylsma, Tune, Brandt, et al. (2003) compared 8 control subjects who were worse at visit 3 on three of five selected neuropsychological tests (decliners) with 24 control subjects who did not show this pattern of decline. The annual mileage at visit 3 was similar for the two groups. Over one-third (37.5%) of the decliners had self-reported crashes between visits 2 and 3, while none of the remaining subjects had. In addition, the number of self-reported near misses was twice as high for the decliners as for the other subjects.

Rizzo, McGehee, Dawson, and Anderson (2001) tested whether licensed drivers with mild cognitive impairment due to Alzheimer's are at greater risk for intersection crashes using the Iowa Driving Simulator (IDS). The results showed that 6 of 18 (33%) of drivers with Alzheimer's experienced crashes compared with none of the 12 nondemented drivers of similar age. The findings were similar to the study cited earlier using rear-end collision avoidance scenarios implemented on the IDS (Rizzo, Reinach, McGehee, et al., 1997). Predictors of crashes in the combined studies included visuospatial impairment, disordered attention, reduced processing of visual motion clues, and overall cognitive decline. Another investigation with Alzheimer's patients (Cox, Quillian, Thornskie, Kovatchev, & Hanna, 1998) compared 29 outpatients with probable Alzheimer's with 21 age-matched controls on the Atari simulator. Driving simulator performance was able to differentiate Alzheimer's patients from control participants and correlated with MMSE scores. Alzheimer's patients drove off the road more often, drove more slowly than the posted speed, applied less brake pressure when trying to stop, spent more time negotiating left-hand turns, and drove more poorly overall than the participants in the control group.

SUMMARY OF OLDER DRIVER SIMULATION STUDIES

The results reported above support the usefulness of high-fidelity simulation and neuropsychological assessment in efforts to standardize the assessment of fitness to drive in older drivers with medical impairments. Although there are methodological weaknesses with many of these studies (e.g., small sample size, reliance on self-report of past automobile crashes, use of noninteractive or nonrealistic simulation systems), they do support the idea that evaluation of driving ability of older people on a driving simulator may be a useful future approach. Driving simulators appear to be sensitive instruments for classifying older drivers who are unsafe to drive, correlating highly with driving skills such as visual search, attention, and choice reaction time. Despite the potential clinical utility of simulators, questions have been raised about the usefulness of simulation with even mildly impaired Alzheimer's patients (see Wild & Cotrell, 2003; Withaar, Brouwer, & van Zomeren, 2000). These criticisms center on the lack of ecological validity and the concern that the novelty of the simulator environment may surpass the capacity of the impaired patient to adapt to it. Although these concerns should not be ignored, they may become less relevant as simulator technology continues to advance and includes enhanced realism (e.g., motion) and simulation of a variety of high-risk driving scenarios.

DRIVING SIMULATION VS. OTHER TYPES OF ASSESSMENT

Judgments about fitness to drive in older drivers should be based on objective, performance-based methods, rather than on age alone. Using age as the sole criterion may unfairly limit mobility in safe older drivers or authorize licensure in adults who are unfit to drive (Rizzo, Jermeland, & Severson, 2002). Several methods of assessing driving ability have been described and researched. These include on-road driving (Hunt, Murphy, Carr, Duchek, Buckles, et al., 1997; Odenheimer, Beaudet, Jette, Albert, Grande, et al., 1994), driving simulator testing (Galski, Ehle, & Williams, 1997; Lee, Lee, & Cameron, 2003), and neuropsychological assessment batteries (Lesikar, Gallo, Rebok, & Keyl, 2002; Marottoli, Richardson, Stowe, Miller, Brass, et al., 1994; Meyers, Volbrecht, & Kaster-Bundergard, 1999; van Zomeren, Brouwer, Rothengater, & Snoek, 1988). In this section, we examine each of these approaches to see which is most feasible and valid for predicting unsafe driving in older drivers.

ON-ROAD DRIVING

Road tests have been considered the standard by which to evaluate driving competence (Freund, Gravenstein, Ferris, & Shaheen, 2002). However, road tests have several limitations since they are often scored subjectively, the road conditions may vary, and the tests may be performed in a car on a driving course that is unfamiliar to the subject. State road tests are designed to ensure that novice drivers know and can apply the rules of the road, not to predict crash involvement in skilled drivers who may have become impaired. Because of their ecological validity relative to other assessment methods, road tests have been advocated by several authors as the preferred method to assess driving competence (Donnelly & Karlinsky, 1990; Kapust & Weintraub, 1992).

SIMULATOR TESTING

Driving simulation appears to be a sensitive method to objectively evaluate driving performance (competence), but the recurrent criticism is that it has not been compared with on-road testing (Freund, Gravenstein, Ferris, & Shaheen, 2002). Driving simulation is widely accepted as safe, reliable, and quantifiable. Unlike on-road testing, simulation is not limited by weather conditions and can easily run multiple variants of the same conditions. The use of contingencies (e.g., paying participants to avoid "crashes") increases realism, and likely the generalizability of simulated performance to that in actual driving situations (Cox, Taylor, & Kovatchev, 1999). Driving simulators also have predictive validity, although their ability to reveal or predict actual on-road performance in older adults, particularly those with cognitive impairments, has not been firmly established.

Testing elderly people in driving simulators does have certain drawbacks. Simulator testing may be too expensive, too unfamiliar, provide unrealistic perceptual information, and have questionable validity. Elderly drivers are more prone to motion sickness, and an older person's ability to act in an unfamiliar technological environment might influence simulated driving performance as a moderating variable (Breker, Rothermel, Verwey, & Henriksson, 2001).

NEUROPSYCHOLOGICAL TESTING

Many studies use neuropsychological testing in conjunction with on-road or driving simulator assessments. Previous research demonstrates that neuropsychological assessments can predict driving status in real-life clinical samples (Galski, Ehle, & Williams, 1997; Meyers, Volbrecht, & Kaster-Bundgaard, 1999). One criticism of the use of neuropsychological tests alone to assess driving-related abilities is their lack of apparent face validity. Another criticism is that the tests are often very time consuming and require considerable training and expertise to reliably administer. Keyl, Rebok, and Gallo (1997) and Lesikar, Gallo, Rebok, and Keyl (2002) have identified a brief battery of paper-and-pencil tests and simple questions about driving habits that can predict unsafe driving behavior in older adults and that are feasible for use by primary care physicians. Computer-based batteries for assessing driving-related skills in older drivers also have been developed for use in clinical care settings and licensing agencies (Dobbs, Heller, & Schopflocher, 1998).

COMPARABILITY OF REAL AND SIMULATED DRIVING

A crucial question is the extent to which driver behavior on advanced simulators relates to actual on-road driving (Blana, 1996). Validity comparisons of on-road vs. simulator studies show similarities on many measures (Reed & Green, 1999; Carsten, Groeger, Blana, & Jamson, 1997; Damkot, 1976; Gawron & Ranney, 1988; Tornros, 1998), but there are few detailed head-to-head comparisons. Many recent studies validated fixed-base driving simulators vs. on-road performance (Blana & Golias, 1999, 2002; Carsten, Groeger, Blana, & Jamson, 1997; Godley, Triggs, &

Fildes, 2002; Reymond, Kemeny, Droulez, & Berthoz, 1999; Tornros, Harms, & Alm, 1997). Several compared subjects in both an instrumented car on a test track or real road and its closely simulated equivalent; correlations were very high for speed choice consistency, mean speed, and lateral road position. Overall, these data suggest the validly of driving simulators in reflecting important aspects of real on-road driving behaviors, (Galley, 1993; Hoffman & Mortimer, 1994).

Only a handful of studies are available that have validated simulators as a method of predicting on-road performance in older adults. In one recent study, Freund and colleagues (2002) compared on-road and simulated driving performance of nine older adults, four of whom were classified as cognitively impaired. Subjects completed a 30-minute driving simulation on the STISIM drive simulator developed by Systems Technology, Inc. and a 30-minute on-road test. The average scores for the simulated and on-road performance were significantly and negatively correlated ($r = -.67$), indicating that fewer errors on the simulator task were related to a higher score on the road test (performance with competency ratings >90%). There was also a strong correlation between hazardous and lethal errors on the simulator and failing the road test ($r = -.83$). In another recent study, Lee, Cameron, & Lee (2003) assessed 129 older drivers on a laboratory-based driving simulator and an on-road test. They found a significant positive correlation between the two indices, with the simulated driving performance index explaining over two-thirds of the variability of the on-road driving performance index, after adjustments for age and gender. Both studies support the validity of the driving simulator for older adults.

USE OF DRIVING SIMULATORS TO RETRAIN OLDER DRIVERS

The positive effects of simulator training on flight safety are well documented and have been demonstrated for several decades using expensive, high-fidelity flight simulators (Hardy & Parasuraman, 1997; Lee & Mollenhauer, 2002). During the past decade technological advances have reduced the costs of graphic hardware and software, allowing high-fidelity simulators to be cost effectively applied to training in other modes of transportation including driving (Allen, Rosenthal, & Parseghian, 1994; Fisher, Laurie, Glaser, Connerney, Pollatsek, et al., 2002). There are several advantages of using simulators in driving training, including training efficiency, safety, standardization and objectivity of driver assessments, and driver-by-driver customization (Lee & Mollenhauer, 2001). The high "face validity" of a realistic, interactive simulated test where results can be reviewed and mistakes explained may be of great value, both in contributing to the effects of retraining and in promoting acceptance and compliance with any subsequent restrictions of driving privilege (Staplin & Hunt, 2003). This is an important advantage since compliance with medical recommendations regarding driving and driving cessation is a major issue facing medical professionals (Bogner, Straton, Gallo, Rebok, & Keyl, 2004; Carr, 2000). Simulators have several other important advantages for driver training, including evaluation of multiple variables with automated monitoring, ability to program driving performance results into several useful formats, and development of reports that can be used to reinforce learning experience on the simulator (Lee & Mollenhauer, 2002).

There is a need for studies comparing simulator training with more traditional forms of driver education and rehabilitation (Hunt, 1993). One type of training that has been the focus of research studies is perceptual training (Ball, 1997; Ball, Beard, Roenker, Miller, & Griggs, 1988). Ball and Owsley (2002) assigned elderly adults who exhibited decreased attentional skills either to a training program to expand the size of their attentional field or to a traditional driving trainer program using a simulator. A third group with normal attentional skills served as the control group. The group that experienced the perceptual training showed improved choice reaction time (RT) and fewer dangerous maneuvers during the driving evaluation. Similar effects were not observed in either the simulator or the control groups. The simulator group improved on three driving performance measures: turning into the correct lane, positioning the vehicle safely at stops, and signaling within 100–150 feet of a turn. Similar effects were not observed in the perceptual training group or the control group. Thus, it seems that training must encompass a variety of techniques to address the global performance of driving. The benefits of this training protocol have been shown to generalize to untrained stimuli and decreased stimulus durations, and to persist for at least one year (Edwards, Wadley, Meyers, Roenker, Cissell, et al., 2002).

Other projects have evaluated educational interventions designed to enhance older driver safety. Recently, Stalvey, and Owsley (2000) and Owsley, Stalvey, and Phillips (2002) reported that an educational intervention for older drivers experiencing decline in visual function and/or UFOV® was effective in modifying self-perceptions about vision and attitudes toward driver safety. Although educational interventions may be offered in classrooms or on a one-on-one basis, advances in technology offer clear advantages for broader dissemination (Ball, Wadley, & Edwards, 2002). For example, free or low-cost driving assessments as well as online courses that can educate older drivers about safe driving practices can both be offered over the Internet.

COMBINING SIMULATOR TECHNOLOGY WITH USE OF FMRI IMAGING AND OTHER TECHNOLOGIES

Understanding the neural basis of performance of real-world, complex, perceptual-motor tasks such as driving is an important goal for future research. This goal is part of an emerging discipline called "neuroergonomics" which comprises two disciplines that themselves are interdisciplinary: neuroscience and ergonomics (Parasuraman, 2003). Neuroergonomics investigates the neural bases of such perceptual and cognitive functions as seeing, hearing, attending, remembering, deciding, and planning in relation to technologies and settings in the real world. It includes the study of many real-world environments, including operating vehicles such as cars, aircraft, trains, and ships.

Simulators offer several important advantages for neuroergonomic studies. They allow for more variability in attentional and behavioral demands presented to subjects and for safe collection of reliable, repeatable, quantitative data. These advantages led recently to simulated driving and flying programs being used in fMRI and electroencephalogram (EEG) research projects (Scheier, 2000; Peres, Van De Moortele, Pierard, Lehericy, Satabin, et al., 2000; Walter, Vetter, Grothe, Wunderlich, Hahn, et al., 2001). For example, Walter and colleagues (2001) studied brain regions correlated with driving using functional magnetic resonance imaging (fMRI) with younger adults who performed a driving simulation task. Participants either steered the car themselves (active driving) or observed while a person outside the scanner was steering the car (passive driving). Results showed common activations in both conditions in occipital and parietal regions bilaterally. Activity specifically associated with driving was found only in the sensorimotor cortex and the cerebellum. Replications of this type of study with older drivers might help identify basic neural mechanisms that underlie safe driving performance. At a practical level, such information might be used to design more effective retraining and rehabilitation programs.

FUTURE DIRECTIONS

In this chapter, we have reviewed and critically evaluated the rapidly expanding use of simulation technology for assessing and training older drivers. Since more older adults will be driving in the next few decades, it is imperative that standardized, objective methods be made available to health professionals and licensing agencies for determining fitness to drive. Although future cohorts of older drivers are expected to be safer than today's older drivers, the cohort effect appears to be small relative to other time-related effects, most notably aging. Therefore, it is expected that older drivers will continue to be a high-risk component of the driving population and will continue to require special consideration in terms of driver training and assessment, driving environment, and vehicular design (Staplin, Lococo, & Sim, 1992; Klavora & Heslegrave, 2002; Eberhard, 1996; Stamatiadis & Deacon, 1995). We have argued that driving simulators hold particular promise for reliably and validly predicting driving safety and for instituting effective crash preventive counter measures in at-risk older drivers.

In response to growing concerns about older driver safety, the American Medical Association has recently developed a guide to help physicians assess and counsel older drivers (Wang & Carr, 2004). Although age is associated with risky driving, it is the conditions associated with aging such as reduced reaction time, decreased attention, and decreased mobility and dexterity that adversely affect driving (Marottoli, Cooney, Wagner, Doucette, & Tinetti, 1994). In addition, many other factors such as medication, neurological disorders such as Alzheimer's disease or Parkinson's disease, brain injury from stroke or head injury, and even lack of sleep may negatively affect driving. Driving simulators, when used in conjunction with other data-gathering techniques, can shed important light on the factors that may make someone a risky driver and that may (or may not) be modifiable through education and training. Two major challenges for future research are to determine more specifically how the brain selects and processes the visual signals from the driving environment and to then use this information to design more targeted crash prevention and crash protection programs. It has been suggested that the study of neuroergonomics is a fertile ground for investigating the relationships between simulated driving behavior and underlying neural mechanisms that may change with age and disease. With this enhanced understanding, researchers should be better prepared to develop intervention programs that can enhance mobility and improve older driver safety.

ACKNOWLEDGMENTS

George W. Rebok is Professor in the Department of Mental Health, The Johns Hopkins University, Bloomberg School of Public Health and School of Medicine, Baltimore, Maryland. Penelope M. Keyl is President, Keyl Associates, East Sandwich, Massachusetts. Requests for reprints should be addressed to G. W. Rebok, Department of Mental Health, Bloomberg School of Public Health, The Johns Hopkins University, 624 North Broadway, Baltimore, MD 21205. E-mail: grebok@jhsph.edu

REFERENCES

Alexander, J., Barham, P., & Black, I. (2002). Factors influencing the probability of an incident at a junction: Results from an interactive driving simulator. *Accident Analysis and Prevention, 34,* 779–792.

Allen, R. W., Rosenthal, T. J., & Parseghian, Z. (1994). *Low cost driving simulation for research, training and screening applications.* Society for Automotive Engineers Congress.

Ball, K. (1997). Enhancing mobility in the elderly: Attentional interventions for driving. In S. M. Dollinger & L. F. DiLalla (Eds.), *Assessment and intervention issues across the life span.* New York: Academic Press.

Ball, K., Beard, B., Roenker, D., Miller, R., & Griggs, D. (1988). Age and visual search: Expanding the Useful Field of View. *Journal of the Optical Society of America, 5,* 2210–2219.

Ball, K., & Owsley, C. (2000). Increasing mobility and reducing accidents of older drivers. In K. W. Schaie & M. Pietrucha (Eds.), *Mobility and transportation in the elderly.* New York: Springer Publishing.

Ball, K., Owsley, C., Sloane, M., Roenker, D., & Bruni, J. (1993). Visual attention problems as a predictor of vehicle accidents among older drivers. *Investigative Ophthalmology & Visual Science, 34,* 3110–3123.

Ball, K., & Rebok, G. (1994). Evaluating the driving ability of older adults. *Journal of Applied Gerontology, 13,* 20–38.

Ball, K. K., Wadley, V. G., & Edwards, J. D. (2002). Advances in technology used to assess and retrain older drivers. *Gerontechnology, 1,* 251–261.

Blana, E. (1996). *Driving simulator validation studies: A literature review.* ITS Working Paper 480.

Blana, E., & Golias, J. (1999). *Behavioral validation of a fixed-base driving simulator.* Paris, France: Driving Simulation Conference.

Blana, E., & Golias, J. (2002). Differences between vehicle lateral displacement on the road and in a fixed-base simulator. *Human Factors, 44,* 303–313.

Bogner, H. R., Straton, J. B., Gallo, J. J., Rebok, G. W., & Keyl, P. M. (2004). The role of physicians in assessing older drivers: Barriers, opportunities, and strategies. *Journal of the American Board of Family Practice, 17,* 38–43.

Breker, S., Rothermel, S., Verwey, W., & Henriksson, P. (2001). *The role of simulation in the assessment of older drivers.* Dortmund, Germany. AGILE Project.

Bylsma, F. W. (1997). Simulators for assessing driving skills in demented patients. *Alzheimer's Disease and Associated Disorders, 11,* 17–20.

Bylsma, F. W., Rebok, G. W., & Keyl, P. M. (1992). Cognitive and simulated driving performance in Alzheimer's disease and normal aging. *Clinical and Experimental Neuropsychology, 14,* 17.

Carr, D. B. (2000). The older adult driver. *American Family Physician, 61,* 141–146, 148.

Carr, D., & Rebok, G. W. (2000). The older driver. In J. J. Gallo, T. Fulmer, G. J. Paveza, & W. Reichel (Eds.), *Handbook of geriatric assessment.* Gaithersburg, MD: Aspen Publishers, Inc.

Carsten, O. M. J., Groeger, J. A., Blana, E., & Jamson, A. H. (1997). *Driver performance in the EPSRC driving simulator: A validation study.* GR/K56162 Final Report. Leeds, England: University of Leeds.

Chaparro, A., Groff, L., Tabor, K., Sifrit, K., & Gugerty, L. J. (1999). *Maintaining situational awareness: The role of visual attention.* Proceedings of the Human Factors and Ergonomics Society 43rd Annual Meeting.

Cox, D. J., Quillian, W. C., Thorndike, F. P., Kovatchev, B. P., & Hanna, G. (1998). Evaluating driving performance of outpatients with Alzheimer's disease. *Journal of the American Board of Family Practice, 11,* 264–271.

Cox, D. J., Taylor, P., & Kovatchev, B. (1999). Driving simulation performance predicts future accidents among older drivers. *Journal of the American Geriatrics Society, 47,* 381–382.

Damkot, D. K. (1976). Alcohol influences: A comparison of on-road driving behavior with instrumented car and laboratory research. *Ergonomics, 19,* 380.

Dobbs, A. R., Heller, R. B., & Schopflocher, D. (1998). A comparative approach to identify unsafe older drivers. *Accident Analysis and Prevention, 30,* 363–370.

Donnelly, R., & Karlinsky, H. (1990). The impact of Alzheimer's disease on driving ability: A review. *Journal of Geriatric Psychiatry and Neurology, 3,* 67–72.

Eberhard, J. (1996). Safe mobility for senior citizens. *International Association for Traffic and Safety Services Research, 20,* 29–37.

Edwards, J. D., Wadley, V. G., Meyers, R. S., Roenker, D. R., Cissell, G. M., & Ball, K. (2002). Transfer of a speed of processing intervention to near and far cognitive functions. *Gerontology, 48,* 329–340.

Emery, C., Robin, J., Knipling, R., Finn, R., & Fleger, S. (1999). *Validation of simulation technology in training, testing, and licensing of tractor-trailer drivers.* U.S. DOT/FHWA Publication No. FHWA-MC-99—060.

Fisher, D. L., Laurie, N. E., Glaser, R., Connerney, K., Pollatsek, A., Duffy, S. A., et al. (2002). Use of a fixed-base driving simulator to evaluate the effects of experience and PC-based risk awareness training on drivers' decisions. *Human Factors, 44,* 287–302.

Freund, B., Gravenstein, S., Ferris, R., & Shaheen, E. (2002). Evaluating driving performance of cognitively impaired and healthy older adults: A pilot study comparing on-road testing and driving simulation. *Journal of the American Geriatrics Society, 50,* 1309–1310.

Galley, N. (1993). The evaluation of the electrooculogram as a psychophysiological measuring instrument in the study of driver behavior. *Ergonomics, 36,* 1063–70.

Galski, T., Ehle, H. T., & Williams, J. B. (1997). Off-road driving evaluations for persons with cerebral injury: A factor analytic study of predriver and simulator testing. *American Journal of Occupational Therapy, 51,* 352–359.

Gawron, V. J., & Ranney, T. A. (1988). The effects of alcohol dosing on driving performance on a closed course and in a driving simulator. *Ergonomics, 31,* 1219–1244.

Gianutsos, R. (1992). The driving advisement system: A computer-augmented quasi-simulation of the cognitive prerequisites for resumption of driving after brain injury. *Assistive Technology, 4,* 70–86.

Godley, S. T., Triggs, T. J., & Fildes, B. N. (2002). Driving simulator validation for speed research. *Accident Analysis and Prevention, 34,* 589–600.

Gruening, J., Bernard, J., Clover, C., & Hoffmeister, K. (1998). *Driving simulation.* SAE Technical Paper No. 980223. Warrendale, MI: Society of Automotive Engineers.

Hakamies-Blomqvist, J., Ostlund, P., Hneroksson, S., (2000). *Elderly drivers in a simulator—a validation study.* VTI Report 464. Linkoping, Sweden.

Hardy, D. J., & Parasuraman, R. (1997). Cognition and flight performance in older pilots. *Journal of Experimental Psychology: Applied, 3,* 313–348.

Hicks, T. G., & Wierville, W. W. (1979). Comparison of five mental workload assessment procedures in a moving base driving simulator. *Human Factors, 21,* 129–143.

Hildreth, E. C., Beusmans, J. M., Boer, E. R., & Royden, C. S. (2000). From vision to action: Experiments and models of steering control during driving. *Journal of Experimental Psychology: Human Perception and Performance, 26,* 1106–1132.

Hoffman, E., & Mortimer, R. (1994). Drivers' estimates of time to collision. *Accident Analysis and Prevention, 26,* 511–520.

Hunt, L. A. (1993). Evaluation and retraining programs for older drivers. *Clinics in Geriatric Medicine, 9,* 439–448.

Hunt, L. A., Murphy, C. F., Carr, D., Duchek, J. M., Buckles, V., & Morris, J. C. (1997). Reliability of the Washington University Road Test. *Archival Neurology, 54,* 707–712.

Jerome, C. J., Ganey, H. C., Mouloua, M., & Hancock, P. A. (2002). Driver workload response to in-vehicle device operations. *International Journal of Occupational Safety and Ergonomics, 8,* 539–546.

Kakaiya, R., Tisovec, R., & Fulkerson, P. (2000). Evaluation of fitness to drive. *Postgraduate Medicine, 107,* 229–236.

Kapust, L., & Weintraub, S. (1992). To drive or not to drive: Preliminary results from road testing of patients with dementia. *Journal of Geriatric Psychiatry and Neurology, 5,* 210–216.

Keyl, P. M., Rebok, G. W., & Gallo, J. J. (1997). *Screening elderly drivers in general medical settings: Toward the development of a valid and feasible assessment procedure.* Final report prepared for the AARP Andrus Foundation, December 1997.

Klavora, P., & Heslegrave, R. J. (2002). Senior drivers: An overview of problems and intervention strategies. *Journal of Aging and Physical Activity, 10,* 322–335.

Lee, H. C., Cameron, D., & Lee, A. H. (2003). Assessing the driving performance of older adult drivers: On-road versus simulated driving. *Accident Analysis and Prevention, 35,* 797–803.

Lee, C., & Mollenhauer, M. (2002). *Driving simulation as a practical and powerful tool in fleet driver assessment and training.* DriveSafetyTM White Paper, November 2002.

Lee, H. C., Lee, A. H., & Cameron, D. (2003). Validation of a driving simulator by measuring the visual attention skill of older adult drivers. *American Journal of Occupational Therapy, 57,* 324–328.

Lesikar, S. E., Gallo, J. J., Rebok, G. W., & Keyl, P. M. (2002). Prospective study of brief neuropsychological measures to assess crash risk in older primary care patients. *Journal of the American Board of Family Practice, 15,* 11–19.

Li, G., Braver, E. R., & Chen, L. H. (2003). Fragility versus excessive crash involvement as determinants of high death rates per vehicle-mile of travel among older drivers. *Accident Analysis and Prevention, 35,* 227–235.

Marottoli, R. A., Cooney, L. M., Wagner, R., Doucette, J., & Tinetti, M. E. (1994). Predictors of automobile crashes and moving violations among elderly drivers. *Annals of Internal Medicine, 121,* 842–846.

Marottoli, R. A., Richardson, E. D., Stowe, M. H., Miller, E.G., Brass, L. M., Coone, et al. (1998). Development of a test battery to identify older drivers at risk for self-reported adverse driving events. *Journal of the American Geriatrics Society, 46,* 562–568.

McGinty, V. B., Shih, R. A., Garrett, E., Calhoun, V. D., Pearlson, G. D. (2001). *Assessment of intoxicated driving with a simulator: A validation study with on-road driving.* International Meeting on Driving Simulation, Iowa City, Iowa.

Meyers, J. E., Volbrecht, M., & Kaster-Bundgaard, J. (1999). Driving is more than pedal pushing. *Applied Neuropsychology, 6,* 154–164.

National Highway Traffic Safety Administration (2001a). *Traffic Safety Facts 2000: A Compilation of Motor Vehicle Crash Data from the Fatality Analysis Reporting System.* Washington, DC: U.S. Department of Transportation.

National Highway Traffic Safety Administration (2001b). *Traffic Safety Facts 2000: Older Population.* Washington, DC: U.S. Department of Transportation.

Odenheimer, G. L., Beaudet, M., Jette, A. M., Albert, M. S., Grande, L., & Minaker, K. L. (1994). Performance-based driving evaluation of the elderly driver: Safety, reliability, and validity. *Journal of Gerontology, 49,* M153–159.

Owsley, C., Ball, K., Sloane, M. E., Roenker, D. L., & Bruni, J. R. (1991). Visual/cognitive correlates of vehicle accidents in older drivers. *Psychology and Aging, 6,* 403–414.

Owsley, C., Stalvey, B. T., & Phillips, J. M. (2003). The effects of an educational intervention in promoting self-regulation among high-risk older drivers. *Accident Analysis and Prevention, 35,* 393–400.

Parasuraman, R. (2003). Neuroergonomics: Research and practice. *Theoretical Issues in Ergonomic Science, 4*(1–2), 5–20.

Peres, M., Van de Moortele, P., Pierard, C., Lehericy, S., Satabin, P., Le Bihan, D., & Guezennec, C. (2000). Functional magnetic resonance imaging of mental strategy in a simulated aviation performance task. *Aviation, Space, and Environmental Medicine, 71,* 1218–1231.

Quillian, W. C., Cox, D. J., Kovatchev, B. P., & Phillips, C. (1999). The effects of age and alcohol intoxication on simulated driving performance, awareness and self-restraint. *Age and Ageing, 28,* 59–66.

Rebok, G. W., Bylsma, F. W., & Keyl, P. M. (1990). The effects of Alzheimer's disease on elderly drivers. *Gerontologist, 30,* 194A.

Rebok, G. W., Keyl, P. M., Bylsma, F. W., Blaustein, M. J., & Tune, L. (1994). The effects of Alzheimer's disease on driving-related abilities. *Alzheimer's Disease and Related Disorders, 8,* 228–240.

Rebok, G. W., Keyl, P. M., Bylsma, F. W., Tune, L., Brandt, J., Teret, S. P. (2003). Cognitive function, driving simulator performance, and crash history in Alzheimer's disease patients and elderly controls. Unpublished manuscript.

Reed, M. P., & Green, P. A. (1999). Comparison of driving performance on-road and in a low-cost simulator using a concurrent telephone dialing task. *Ergonomics, 42,* 1015–1037.

Reymond, G., Kemeny, A., Droulez, J., & Berthoz, A. (1999). *Contribution of a motion platform to kinesthetic restitution in a driving simulator.* Driving Simulation Conference, Paris, France.

Rizzo, M., Jermeland, J., & Severson, J. (2002). Instrumented vehicles and driving simulation. *Gerontechnology, 1,* 291–296.

Rizzo, M., Reinach, S., McGehee, D. V., & Dawson, J. (1997). Simulated car crashes and crash predictors in drivers with Alzheimer's disease. *Archives of Neurology, 54,* 545–551.

Rizzo, M., McGehee, D. V., Dawson, J. D., & Anderson, S. N. (2001). Simulated car crashes at intersections in drivers with Alzheimer's disease. *Alzheimer's Disease and Associated Disorders, 15,* 10–20.

Schier, M. A. (2000). Changes in EEG alpha power during simulated driving: A demonstration. *International Journal of Psychophysiology, 37,* 155–162.

Stalvey, B. T., & Owsley, C. (2000). Self-perceptions and current practices of high-risk older drivers: Implications for driver safety interventions. *Journal of Health Psychology, 5,* 441–456.

Stamatiadis, N., & Deacon, J. A. (1995). Trends in highway safety: Effects of an aging population on accident propensity. *Accident Analysis and Prevention, 27,* 443–459.

Staplin, L. (1995). Simulator and field measures of driver age differences in left-turn gap judgments. *Transportation Research Record, 1485,* 49–55.

Staplin, L., & Hunt, L. (2003). Driver programs. In *Transportation in an Aging Society: A Decade of Experience.* Washington, DC: Transportation Research Board, National Academy of Sciences/National Research Council.

Staplin, L., Lococo, K., & Sim, J. (1992). *Traffic maneuver problems of older drivers: Final technical report.* Federal Highways Administration Report No. FHWA-RD-92—092, McLean, Virginia.

Stutts, J. C., Stewart, J. R., & Martell, C. M. (1998). Cognitive test performance and crash risk in an older driver population. *Accident Analysis and Prevention, 30,* 337–346.

Tornros, J. (1998). Driving behavior in a real and a simulated road tunnel: A validation study. *Accident Analysis and Prevention, 30,* 497–503.

Tornros, J., Harms, L., & Alm, H. (1997). The VTI simulator: Validation studies. DSC '97 Driving Simulation Conference. Lyons, France.

U.S. Bureau of the Census(2003). Projections of the total resident population by 5-year age groups, and sex with special age categories: Middle Series, 2025–2045. Available at www.census.gov/population/projections/nation/summary/np-t3-f.txt

Van Zomeren, A. H., Brouwer, W. H., Rothengatter, J. A., & Snoek, J. W. (1988). Fitness to drive a car after recovery from severe head injury. *Archives of Physical Medicine and Rehabilitation, 69,* 697–705.

Verwey, W. B. (2000). On-line driver workload estimation. Effects of road situation and age on secondary task measures. *Ergonomics, 43,* 187–209.

Wallace, R. B. (1997). Cognitive change, medical illness, and crash risk among older drivers: An epidemiological consideration. *Alzheimer's Disease and Associated Disorders, 11,* 31–37.

Walter, H., Vetter, S. C., Grothe, J., Wunderlich, A. P., Hahn, S., & Spitzer, M. (2001). The neural correlates of driving. *Neuroreport, 12,* 1763–1767.

Wang, C. C., & Carr, D. B. (2004). Older driver safety: a report from the older drivers project. *Journal of the American Geriatrics Society, 52,* 143–149.

Weir, D. H., & Clark, A. J. (1996). A survey of mid-level driving simulators. *Society of Automotive Engineers and Transportation, 104,* 86.

Wild, K., & Cotrell, V. (2003). Identifying driving impairment in Alzheimer disease: A comparison of self and observer reports versus driving evaluation. *Alzheimer's Disease and Associated Disorders, 17,* 27–34.

Withaar, F. K., Brouwer, W. H., & Van Zomeren, A. H. (2000). Fitness to drive in older adults with cognitive impairment. *Journal of the International Neuropsychological Society, 6,* 480–490.

14

The Dr. Tong Louie Living Laboratory: A Unique Facility for the Research and Development of Assistive Technology

James Watzke

SCIENTIFIC AND HISTORICAL CONTEXT

Starting in the late 1960s there were numerous significant efforts to promote the importance of person-environment (P-E) transactions upon the affective, behavioral, and/or functional outcomes of older adults (e.g., Barker, 1968; Pastalan & Carson, 1970; Craik, 1970; Lawton & Simon, 1968). Undoubtedly, the most articulate proponent of P-E modeling was Powell Lawton, who developed the Environmental Docility Hypothesis that stated "the less competent the individual, the greater the impact of environmental factors on that individual" (Lawton & Simon, 1968, p. 11). Later, Lawton proposed the Environmental Proactivity Hypothesis, which conversely suggests that "as personal competence increases, the variety of environmental resources that can be used in satisfaction of the persons' needs increases" (Lawton, 1990, p. 639). These theoretical generalizations are important for they became the basis for a myriad of other important concepts such as "person-environment fit," prosthetic environments," "user-friendly products," "adaptive housing," and "supportive environments for persons with special needs." To understand the legitimacy of Lawton's theories, one need only observe a person in a wheelchair attempt to use a conventional bathroom, or a five-foot, two-inch 85-year-old with arthritis prepare a meal in her standard kitchen using standard appliances.

Although a strong theoretical foundation was in place, the fields of Gerontology, Human Factors, Environmental Psychology, Architecture, Interior Design, Rehabilitation Medicine, and Biomedical Engineering continued to produce a shortfall of rigorous data showing how, and to what extent, older adults and persons with disabilities respond to and negotiate the demands of everyday tasks in their environments, including their interactions with everyday consumer products and/or assistive technologies (e.g., Chapanis, 1974; Koncelik, 1977; Fozard, 1981; Raschko, 1982; Faletti, 1984; Czaja, 1990). The Living Lab was developed as a modest attempt to counteract this knowledge gap, and was guided by a comprehensive paradigm for human factors research for an aging population (Czaja, 1990).

To summarize, at the conceptual stage, three types of scientific data were envisioned to be produced in the Lab for older adults and persons with disabilities, namely: 1) task analysis data of activities of daily living; 2) person-environment data for the improved design of residential and/or institutional interiors, and 3) human factors data related to the proper evaluation of specific products or technologies. As discussed below, some of these perceived research domains have been more fruitful (for the Lab) than others.

FACILITY DEVELOPMENT CHALLENGES

The initial conceptual proposal for the Living Lab was written in 1991 (Watzke, 1991). As with any new initiative within an academic institution, we were required to develop and prove a case for the Living Lab. This entailed: 1) review of existing (or competing) full-scale simulation laboratories and/or research groups; 2) execution of some "proof of concept" research; and 3) acquisition of funding. During this phase, research staff contacted and assessed numerous settings across Canada, the United States, and Europe that were believed to engage in full-scale simulation activities AND had an interest in gerontology, rehabilitation, and/or improving "age- and disability-sensitive" design of environments or products (Watzke, 1991). This exploration convinced us that the facility we had envisioned was needed and viable for Western Canada, and British Columbia.

As part of a strategy to procure required space and funding, some "proof of concept" research was conducted to demonstrate the potential contribution of such a facility to gerontechnology and related fields. Accordingly, staff convinced a local commercial real estate corporation to donate approximately 800 square feet of prime downtown Vancouver office space for a funded research project that required a full-scale residential simulation. The project focused on a human factors evaluation of a prototype portable electronic environmental control device (Watzke & Birch, 1994; Watzke, 1997). Of most importance, this opportunity allowed staff to: 1) revise and refine our concept for the Living Lab; 2) showcase a full-scale model of the envisioned Lab for potential donors, funders, and partners; and 3) show how the full-scale simulation facility enhanced our ability to produce publishable applied research.

As might be expected, fundraising was the most critical and time consuming need and included the following ingredients over a six year period:

1. The Simon Fraser University Development Office agreed to make the Living Lab a high priority for their fund raising. After two or three years of work, they identified a significant private donor (Dr. Tong Louie) and obtained a match to his gift from the Government of British Columbia. This resulted in a permanent Lab Endowment.

2. One additional key academic partner (British Columbia Institute of Technology-BCIT) and one community-based partner (Neil Squire Foundation) were engaged for the initiative. The former provided the Lab with permanent space in a new BCIT building. Both partners had the technical and research staffs to enhance the overall capability of the Lab.

3. The momentum of number one and two above allowed the new facility to capture significant funds for needed equipment, infrastructure, research contracts and grants, and increased staffing (from both private and public funding sources). To date, the above sources of funding total approximately CAN $1.75 million.

PHYSICAL STRUCTURE

The Lab comprises three primary spaces, as described below.

EXPERIMENTAL STUDIO

Resembling a movie set, this 1000-square-foot open area allows researchers to simulate, in full scale, the features, products, or environments needed for a given project. For example, we have simulated multiple kitchens, bathrooms, a grocery store and pharmacy counters, workstations, and a full one-bedroom apartment. Incorporating moveable walls, a ceiling grid, and a raised subfloor to allow maximum flexibility in simulation options, the Experimental Studio is the Lab's the central location for data collection.

VIEWING THEATRE

Researchers and visitors can unobtrusively observe and respond to activity in the Experimental Studio from the adjacent Viewing Theatre. Similar to the viewing theatres found in the surgery units of teaching hospitals, it contains one-way glass, TV monitors, and personal computers interfaced with the Lab's Data Acquisition and Analysis Centre.

DATA ACQUISITION AND ANALYSIS CENTRE

Using fully interactive and networked personal computers, portable audio and video technology, a sophisticated motion analysis system (PEAK), and an automated remote audience response technology system, the Lab can capture a variety of human, product, device, and environmental performance data. Typical methods employed are behavioural observation, self-report questionnaires, task analysis, and three-dimensional biomechanical motion analysis.

LAB STAFFING & EXPERTISE

A key factor to the Lab's success is its access to and utilization of multidisciplinary teams. For every project, a designated Project Leader assembles the appropriate team members. The Living Lab benefits significantly from being part of a larger 55-person research center, the BCIT Technology Centre. BCIT is the largest polytechnic institute in Western Canada. The Living Lab falls under the subgroup of the Technology Centre called the Health Technology Research Group (HTRG). Presently, the HTRG employs 11 full-time personnel with expertise in architecture, assistive and medical device design, behavioural psychology, biomedical engineering, clinical engineering, electrical engineering, environmental psychology, gerontology, health care epidemiology, human factors/ergonomics, human kinetics, industrial design, marketing, mechanical engineering, plastics, product evaluation (usability testing), prototype production, prosthetics & orthotics, robotics, and software design and evaluation. In addition, the Lab has access to various faculty members across BCIT, which represents over 200 separate training programs. Core and full-time Lab staff that work in the Lab on a full-time basis include a research head (the author), two research associates, and a part-time administrative assistant. In sum, the Lab's facilities and staffing resources provide a unique and powerful resource for behaviour observation, human factors analysis, physiological measurement, and product evaluation.

LAB OPERATION, RESEARCH APPROACH, AND SERVICES

As Lab activities increased, policies and procedures for access and utilization were necessary. Therefore, a comprehensive, legally binding collaboration agreement stipulates the procedures and regulations governing all partners and users of the Lab. It delineates how Lab access and research activities are to be prioritized, how the endowment and other Lab funding is to be spent, and who is responsible for the daily operation (and expenses) of the Lab. An executive steering committee oversees compliance with the collaboration agreement and addresses any other operational needs of the Lab. For BCIT, all staff utilized for Living Lab projects are under a "salary recovery model," i.e., staff time is accounted for and wherever possible paid for from existing research contracts or grants. The BCIT Technology Centre and Lab Endowment cover any nonrecovered portions of core staff salaries.

As part of the polytechnic institute, BCIT staff working in the Living Lab are expected to focus on applied research and development (R&D) (as opposed to a basic research mandated at many traditional university research settings), and wherever possible to promote industry and economic development and increased quality of life for citizens of British

Columbia and Canada. Based on our mandate and resources, our work has been most successful within two domains. Under the first domain, technical staff develop (design, fabricate prototypes, and produce) all types of medical and assistive devices including: (a) safer and more effective acute care and diagnostic technologies, including emergency room, surgical, and diagnostic tools; (b) tools and workstations designed to reduce injury to health care workers; and (c) assistive technologies designed to meet the growing demand for increased independence for older adults and persons with disabilities. We embrace a broad definition of assistive technology, i.e., any product, system, or environmental feature that can help the individual to accomplish any daily living or work tasks.

Second, we have the facilities, expertise, and interest in testing and evaluating systems, products (including assistive technology), small-scale environments, and procedures to ensure the safety and optimal performance of such devices used by assorted users, e.g., older adults, persons with disabilities, and health care professionals. It is in this domain that the Living Lab plays a primary role, e.g., by developing usability protocols, obtaining ethics approvals, conducting clinical trials, and executing feasibility and market research on various devices and products. Where appropriate, researchers working in both domains have developed and utilize a quality system that follows International Standards Organization (ISO) protocols, U.S. Food and Drug Administration (FDA) design controls, and Health Canada guidelines. This ensures our work meets regulatory standards in Canada, the U.S., and Europe.

Living Lab external research funding typically comes from a blend of external competitive grants and industry-based contracts. Grant sources have included private and not-for-profit foundations and agencies, provincial programs, and federal agencies or institutes. Private industry contracts have typically come from medium and small Canadian companies. Project fees vary based on need and scope. The next section demonstrates how the Lab's approach has materialized in actual projects.

PAST, CURRENT, AND FUTURE PROJECTS

The following is a brief description of selected past, current, and future Living Lab projects, because they are relevant to assistive technology and the themes of this book. First, some basic principles apply to most projects executed in the Lab: 1) wherever feasible, we recruit (and pay an honorarium) to research participants who are the intended or actual users of the devices or products being studied; 2) the Lab follows strict ethical guidelines as stipulated by a Canadian-wide council on research ethics; and 3) several Lab projects have proprietary elements, requiring research staff to maintain the confidentiality of any intellectual property associated with a project. This also limits our ability to describe and publish information about selected projects.

Devices To Prevent Injury to Home Support Workers

In British Columbia, home support workers experience the highest injury rates among health care workers, especially musculoskeletal injuries (MSIs) to their backs (Workers Compensation Board of BC-WCB, 2000). Under a research program of the WCB, our staff has been awarded a series of grants to address this problem. In the first study, four low-tech devices were selected that were hypothesized to reduce MSIs for home support workers as they transfer and lift. The devices were: 1) transfer belt; 2) raised toilet seat; 3) portable bathtub grab bar; and 4) portable bath bench. A full-scale typical residential bathroom was simulated in the Lab, actual home support workers served as subjects (n = 21), and another participant was trained to act as an elderly client in need of bathroom transfers (see Figure 14.1).

The home support worker and client dyads performed a protocol of several toilet and bathtub transfers using the four study aids, as well as a manual (no aid) condition. Among other methods, a 3-D motion analysis system (PEAK) was used to perform biomechanical analyses to estimate the relative risk for back injury to the home support workers. Findings led researchers to conclude that none of the studied devices reduced the risk of injury to the home support worker (Watzke, Paris-Seeley, & Raschke, 1999; Paris-Seeley, Raschke, Watzke, Jones, & Halsted, 2000; Raschke, Paris-Seeley, Watzke, Jones, Groves, et al., 2001; Heacock, Paris-Seeley, Raschke, & Watzke, 2002).

Based on these results, we continued the research convinced that the best injury prevention strategy is to make sure home support workers do no home-based client transfers without the use of a mechanical or electrical lift. We received another grant to develop such a lift that would meet the performance requirements of the commercially available electrical lifts, but would be portable and less costly. We have entered into a partnership with a company that produces and distributes client lifts. The partnership allowed us to conduct clinical trials with the prototype lift in order to properly assess (in actual clients' homes) the performance

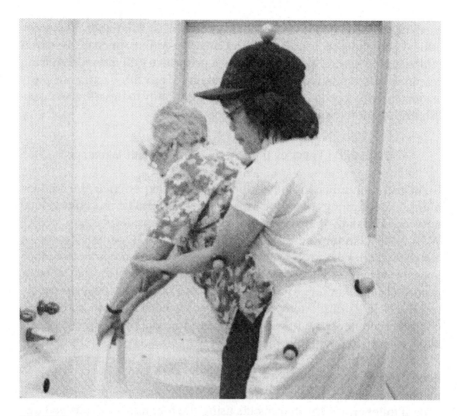

FIGURE 14.1 Transfer aid study of an in-home patient transfer. A home support worker is executing a bathtub transfer with a trained senior aged client in the "transfer aid study." The round reflector balls (markers) are placed on participants' selected joints, allowing researchers to estimate risk of injury using the 3-D biomechanical motion analysis system and appropriate biomechanical calculations.

and commercial viability of the lift (competing lifts are included in the field studies). If the clinical trials are successful, the commercial partner will assist with the commercialization of the lift, including protection of intellectual property, liability, and marketing challenges.

IMPROVING THE USABILITY AND ACCESSIBILITY OF ELECTRONIC DAILY LIVING DEVICES

Since the initial proof of concept research for the Living Lab (Watzke & Birch, 1994), together with our partner the Neil Squire Foundation, we have engaged in several studies to develop and improve the usability and accessibility of electronic daily living devices, such as debit card handsets, and personal digital assistants. The Neil Squire R&D Group (www.neilsquire.ca) has a 15-year track record of developing technologies for persons with significant physical disabilities (Birch, Watzke, & Bolduc, 1995). A mutually beneficial relationship has developed over the years, especially toward the exploration of what we call the "crossover potential" of some of Neil Squire's assistive technologies. A good example of this type of research focused on an automated integrated environmental control device that was developed for younger persons with spinal cord injury, but was thought to be relevant to the lives of older adults with disabilities (Watzke & Birch, 1994; Watzke, 1997).

Our methodology researching electronic daily living aids in the Living Lab often includes a "micro" and "macro" approach. First we study the micro dimensions of a given device or prototype (e.g., LCD screen qualities, software menu, keypad configuration and function, etc.). Then we focus on relevant macro dimensions such as ambient lighting and noise, apparatus to hold the handset, accessibility of countertops for wheelchairs, store clerk behaviour, etc.

Over time, we have learned that conducting R&D on electronic devices for these groups presents significant challenges such as: 1) the quickly changing product development landscape inherent with most electronic consumer products, i.e., keeping up with the changing technology and earning the right to have input into the product design cycle early enough; and 2) convincing manufacturers to take a genuine interest in the inherently small market represented by actual consumers of such devices who are older adults or persons with disabilities.

Consequently, we have refined our strategy to focus on improving the usability and accessibility of existing devices by improving their interfaces, i.e., to make them more user friendly for older adults and persons with disabilities. We are currently engaged (with Neil Squire) in two projects using this approach. The first utilizes a detailed human factors protocol to study alternative interfaces (e.g., track balls, electronic head pointers) to explore how one might improve the accessibility of commercially available personal digital assistants (PDAs) for persons with spinal cord injury (n = 31). This project continues our work in the Lab on the topic of environmental control devices. Neil Squire received a Federal Grant from the Canadian Institutes of Health Research to "prove the principle" of this accessible PDA work. This will allow researchers to explore the commercial potential of the original concept or elements involved in the research.

In the second project, we completed a comprehensive set of in-Lab and field studies to provide the Canadian Bankers Association with "performance recommendations" on how to improve the accessibility of point of sale (debit card) devices for persons with disabilities. Participants (n = 80) included persons with vision impairments, hand and mobility impairments, and a subgroup of older adults. One probable outcome of this project is for the findings to be utilized in a process to create a Canadian national standard of accessibility for such devices (e.g., Canadian Standards Association, 2001).

IMPROVING DEVICES, PRODUCTS, AND WORKSTATIONS USED BY INSTITUTION-BASED HEALTH CARE WORKERS

Unfortunately, several health care worker groups in addition to the one described above have increased risk for injuries (Workers Compensation Board, 2000). BCIT and Living Lab researchers have been contracted to address technological or product improvements and/or solutions to several injury scenarios being experienced by such health care workers. For example: 1) nurses experience MSIs and other hazards in the process of crushing pills and using ineffectively designed medication carts, both important activities on any in-patient long-term care setting; 2) ultrasound technicians (sonographers) report significant work-related injuries due to the complicated and demanding tasks required in ultrasound data collections; and 3) laboratory technicians engaged in "pipetting," experience high rates of MSIs in specimen processing for various laboratory tests. A similar pattern led to our involvement in each of these areas: 1) worker injury claims were being reported across several institutional work settings for the same tasks and worker groups; 2) authorities responsible for the health and well-being of such workers recognized the problems and wanted solutions; and 3) our staff has a reputation for developing, evaluating, and helping apply technological solutions to such problems, especially for health care personnel. Our strategy in each project was also similar. First we studied the nature of the problem, and assessed current devices, products, workstations, and work task practices involved in each scenario. Next, we generally applied R&D expertise to develop and/or improve one or more of the product or technological elements our analyses told us might reduce injury. In these examples, this included designing and prototyping a better automated "pill crusher" as well as designing and prototyping a better medication cart, which is almost always used in tandem with pill crushing technology.

For the ultrasound sonographers and pipetter lab technicians, we did significant R&D leading to improved alternatives. At some point all four projects were simulated and evaluated in the Living Lab, using actual health care workers as participants, and using a variety of human factors and qualitative data collection methods. After the Lab evaluations, the products or workstations are typically placed in the field for further testing and clinical trials. Often in parallel to the Lab and field studies, staff explore any intellectual property that may be associated with each of the projects, as well as searching for potential commercial partners to investigate the viability/feasibility of taking any or some portion of the work to market (see final section for further discussion on this topic).

STUDENT PROGRAMS TO PROMOTE INTEREST IN THE CREATION OF ASSISTIVE TECHNOLOGY: SOLUTIONS AND PROTOGÉ

These two programs have a several year history in British Columbia. In SOLUTIONS, typically each year 50–60 student groups from various post-secondary academic programs (mostly industrial design, occupational therapy, and engineering) agree to focus their course projects on the conceptualization and in some cases, prototype creation of an original assistive device. SOLUTIONS culminates in an annual exposition held at a local rehabilitation center, where a wide spectrum of clients and staff gather to give the students valued feedback (and inspiration) on their projects.

In the second program, PROTOGÉ, each year an advisory committee identifies approximately 12 of the SOLUTIONS projects deemed to have "the most commercial potential." In this voluntary program, for the entire academic year students participate in a "mentoring program" where, with the help of senior level professionals (many from private assistive technology industry or clinical settings), they execute tasks to explore the commercial potential of their prototypes. Many of those tasks focus on marketing issues (e.g., competitive product analyses, market-share projections, user testing, and financing) since that is the training the students are least likely to receive in their academic programs. To date three PROTOGÉ projects have acquired patents, and a few participants have gained employment at mentors' companies or in the medical or assistive device industry. For more detail about these programs, see Watzke (2002a).

Technology for Caregivers of Persons with Dementia

A final category of assistive technology research the Lab conducts is best termed "market research." Canada has several government-based programs mandated to help companies develop new technologies or products. Many require companies to conduct external market research on their concept or product as a condition of receiving funding. For example, we recently conducted market research for a company specializing in health and behavioural management systems for persons with Alzheimer's. We engaged faculty from our business school to do the secondary research (e.g., competitive economic analyses, distribution strategies), while the Living Lab team simulated the needed technology or prototype system to facilitate usability and focus group events (primary, original data collection). In this case, 21 caregivers of persons with Alzheimer's were invited to the Lab and participated in a full-scale product simulation/demonstration and market research data collection protocol. Between the two types of data, we provided the client with a confidential and comprehensive market assessment and a marketing strategy for their proposed new product or system.

LESSONS LEARNED & FUTURE ACTIVITIES

The first five years of operation of the Living Lab provide several observations and insights. First, two major research areas expected to be successful in the Lab have not materialized: 1) studies of activities of daily living for older adults, and 2) studies of residential environments or interiors. We are not certain why these research domains have not fared well in the Lab, but for the former, it might be hypothesized that under restricted federal budgets, most health funding is focused on delivery of health care services as opposed to health research. When one reviews recent Canadian federal and provincial health research funding guidelines, relatively little is directed at geriatric rehabilitation, community-based health research, and/or R&D on health technologies. Unfortunately, these are the health research domains that Living Lab is best suited for. Regarding residential and/or environmental design research in the Lab, there is no longer a significant public funding envelope in Canada for such research, e.g., on accessible, barrier-free, and/or adaptive residential design. We have also learned that private housing developers and/or public housing agencies are unlikely to invest in full-scale research on age and disability sensitive design.

Another important lesson learned is how challenging it is to bring products or devices to market, and ideally enjoy some margin of commercial success; few assistive technology products that reach prototype stage actually become commercialized (Fernie, 1997;, 2002b). We are currently focusing on being associated with more products that we hope will make it to market. Toward this goal we are also seeking additional funding to hire a full-time "technology transfer manager" to augment our existing skills set.

On the positive side, it is now evident that research and development activities focused on product-user interfaces with a variety of medical and assistive devices are fruitful for the facility. Several such projects were described above. We have also learned that research on products and technologies that help prevent injury to assorted health care personnel is also well suited for the Living Lab. Possible explanations for these positive outcomes are many. In both domains, economic forces are driving the need for R&D. Companies are trying to produce economically viable health industry products, and although an inverse economics is operating in the case of health care worker injuries, all stakeholders (employers, workers, and workers compensation agencies) are motivated to reduce the costs associated with injured workers.

Although difficult to measure, the benefits of the Lab's full-scale simulation Experimental Studio cannot be overestimated. Research staff believe our ability to mock up even modest environmental contexts for the assorted products and devices studied has provided invaluable ecological and technical validity for several projects. This is further enhanced because, by policy, Living Lab research requires actual or intended users to be involved in the evaluation of the devices, products, or systems under study. Clearly, in-Lab research is not a substitute for more ecologically valid field research. Thus, the Lab research is but one step that allows our researchers to then safely take devices or products into the field, where further clinical and test trials can be executed. Also the multidisciplinary skills sets of our "in-house" team are critical to our R&D successes. These diverse professionals allow us to execute diverse health technology projects and apply critical creative problem-solving energies (without worrying about being charged for every hour spent discussing a project or problem).

Future projects planned for the Lab will continue to build on our track record. We have been asked to partner with a Finnish research group to help them execute North American user testing for a prototype "intelligent moving aid" for the elderly. We also recently received a contract with Health Canada and the Canadian Standards Association to conduct original pilot research to determine the viability and best methods of having an age- and disability-friendly consumer-product labeling program in Canada. Finally, we will soon manage a health promotion initiative that will create the first Canadian national television-based public service announcement (PSA) to promote positive use of assistive technology by Canadian seniors and veterans. This unique project is one of many under a federal falls prevention initiative sponsored by Health Canada and Veterans Affairs Canada.

ACKNOWLEDGMENTS

James Watzke is Director, Health Technology Research Group, Technology Centre, British Columbia Institute of Technology, Vancouver, British Columbia, Canada, V6B 3H6. The author gratefully acknowledges the contributions to and assistance with this chapter by Christine Flegal, Project Leader, Living Laboratory.

REFERENCES

Barker, R. G. (1968). *Ecological Psychology: Concepts and methods for studying the environment of human behavior.* Stanford, CA: Stanford University Press.

Birch, G., Watzke, J. R., & Bolduc, C. (1995). Research and development of adaptive equipment for persons with significant disabilities and the elderly: Activities conducted by the Neil Squire Foundation. *Technology and Disability, 4,* 169–173.

Canadian Standards Association (2001). *Barrier-free design for automated banking machines.* Can/CSA B651, 1–01. Toronto: Author

Chapanis, A. (1974). Human engineering environments for the aged. *Applied Ergonomics, 5*(2), 75–80.

Craik, K. H. (1970). Environmental Psychology. In T. M. Newcomb (Ed.), *New directions in psychology.* New York: Holt, Rinehart, & Winston.

Czaja, S. J. (Ed.) (1990). *Human factors research needs for an aging population.* Washington DC: National Academy Press.

Faletti, M. V. (1984). Human factors research and functional environments for the aged. In I. Altman, J. E. Wohlwill, & M. P. Lawton (Eds.), *Elderly people and the environment.* New York: Plenum Press.

Fernie, G. (1997). Bringing the product from the design concept to the marketplace. In G. Gutman, (Ed.), *Technology innovation for an aging society: Blending research, public and private sectors.* Vancouver: Gerontology Research Centre, Simon Fraser University.

Fozard, J. L. (1981). Person-environment relationships in adulthood: Implications for human factors engineering. *Human Factors, 23,* 7–28.

Heacock, H., Paris-Seeley, N., Raschke, S., & Watzke, J. (2002, October). *Lift devices to reduce musculoskeletal injuries among home support workers in British Columbia.* Proceedings of the 17th Annual Meeting of the Association of Canadian Ergonomists, Banff, Alberta.

Koncelik, J. (1977). Human factors and environmental design for aging: Physiological change and sensory loss and design criteria. In T. Byerts, S. Howell, and L. Pastalan (Eds.), *Environmental Context of Aging.* New York: Van Nostrand Reinhold.

Lawton, M. P., & Simon, B. (1968). The ecology of social relationships in housing for the elderly. *Gerontologist, 8,* 108–115.

Lawton, M. P. (1990). Residential environment and self-directedness among older people. *American Psychologist, 45*(5), 638–640.

Paris-Seeley, N. J ., Raschke, S. U., Watzke, J. W., Jones, Y., & Halsted, N. (March 2000). *Evaluation of portable transfer devices to reduce the risk of musculoskeletal injury (MSI) to home care workers and development of performance requirements for such devices.* Final Report to Workers Compensation Board of British Columbia. Available at www.worksafebc.com

Pastalan, L. A., & Carson, D. H. (Eds.) (1970). *Spatial behaviour of older people.* Ann Arbor: University of Michigan Press.

Raschke, S. U., Paris-Seeley, N. J., Watzke, J. W., Jones, Y., Groves, M., & Halsted, N. (2001). Evaluation of portable, low-cost transfer devices used by home health care workers. *Orthopadei-Technik Quarterly,* English Edition, 111.

Raschko, B. (1982). *Housing interiors for the disabled and elderly.* New York: Van Nostrand Reinhold.

Watzke, J. (1991). *The Living Laboratory: A proposed centre for the study of effective environmental design for older and/or disabled adults.* Unpublished paper, Gerontology Research Centre, Simon Fraser University, Vancouver, British Columbia.

Watzke, J., & Birch, G. (1994). Older adults' responses to automated environmental control devices. In G. Gutman & A. Wister (Eds.), *Progressive accommodation for seniors: Interfacing shelter and services.* Vancouver: Gerontology Research Centre, Simon Fraser University.

Watzke, J. (1997). Older adults' responses to an automated integrated environmental control device: The case of the Remote Gateway. *Technology and Disability, 7,* 103–114.

Watzke, J., Paris-Seeley, N., & Raschke, S. (1999, November). *Evaluation of portable transfer devices to reduce musculoskeletal injury (MSI) to home care workers.* Paper presented at the 52nd Annual Meeting of the Gerontology Society of America, San Francisco, California.

Watzke, J. (2002a, October). *The Dr. Tong Louie Living Lab: Recent activities involving human factors.* Proceedings of the 17th Annual Meeting of the Association of Canadian Ergonomists, Banff, Alberta. Watzke, J. (2002b). Assistive technology for older adults: Challenges of product development and evaluation. *Gerontechnology, 2*(1), 68–76.

Workers Compensation Board of British Columbia (2000). *Health care industry: Focus report on occupational injury.* Available at www.worksafebc.com

15

New Participative Tools in Product Development for Seniors

Hans-Liudger Dienel,
Alexander Peine, and
Heather Cameron

INTRODUCTION

In 1997 Daniel Goleman published a book on "emotional intelligence." Replacing the classical paradigm that intelligence could be measured in terms of cognitive and logical activities Goleman proposed a view of intelligence that emphasized the role of emotions in the way we value things and decide about our subsequent course of action. Consistent with this principle of emotional intelligence, our view on technologies and technological designs should also change. It should no longer be seen as purely driven by specific tasks, tools and traditional human factors considerations, but also by individual attributes such as specific hopes, wishes, fears, and attitudes. This is the core principle of a German research group that develops everyday technology for senior households. The group seeks to develop emotional technologies.

We assert that current senior-appropriate technology is far from being emotional technology in a positive way. Rather, it is often stigmatized as technology for the disabled or as technology to compensate for shortcomings with regard to physical dexterity, eyesight, concentration, and coordination, among other factors. In other words, senior-appropriate technology is currently determined by all kinds of physical or mental deficits usually attributed to seniors. We think that it is time to change this erroneous belief system. Due to our aging society it is increasingly important to provide product developers with a methodology that encourages senior-appropriate product design that meets the diverse specific demands and potentials of elderly individuals. This is what we would call "emotional assistive technology": products that enhance seniors' power rather than merely compensate for their shortcomings.

We describe this methodology to develop emotional assistive technology in three steps. First, we show how three different levels of objectives characterize our methodology: a normative level, a strategic level, and an operational level. Second, several dimensions form each of these levels. We identify seven dimensions that must be explored in more detail to understand how the objective of emotional technologies can be accomplished. Third, we introduce specific results of our multidisciplinary research conducted at the Technical University Berlin. We have developed and honed our methodology within the "Sentha" (*Seniorengerechte Technik im häuslichen Alltag*—Everyday Technology for the Elderly) project. This methodology is not necessarily limited to the development of assistive technologies, but can also be applied to fields of product development for other target groups and technological fields. We conclude this chapter by highlighting research activities necessary to optimize this methodology.

THE CORNERSTONES OF THE METHODOLOGY

First, our approach attempts to counter two gerontological design dogmata: the concepts of "barrier free products" and "design for all." Rejecting these concepts as not useful, we then developed a hierarchy of objectives to replace the old standards. This hierarchy is based on a set of normative objectives. Normative objectives can be understood as fundamental objectives: questioning their importance would only lead to the conviction that they simply are important (Keeney, 1992). Normative objectives constitute the basic principles upon which we act in our private or professional life.

Normative objectives do not necessarily enable the product developer to derive directives for concrete courses of action. Rather, they must first be translated into strategic objectives that provide guidance for action in a narrower range of circumstances. Although they might still be quite generic, they provide guidelines tailored to a specific context. For the purposes of this chapter, it is important to understand the hierarchical relationship between normative and strategic objectives: strategic objectives are means objectives, e.g., objectives that aim to fulfill other objectives (for example, if we strive for a reduction of CO_2 emissions in order to mitigate the greenhouse effect, this is the ends objective.)

Strategic objectives, in turn, do not elaborate on the process by which they can be accomplished. Hence, it is most crucial to translate strategic objectives into operational objectives (Quade, 1985). In other words, it is important to define objectives that give concrete procedural guidelines in a certain situation. Operational objectives are hierarchically subordinate to strategic objectives. They allow meeting the strategic objectives and, thereby, the normative objectives to be met.

The methodology described in this chapter enables designers to develop products that appeal to seniors in the sense that they feel satisfied to purchase and use them. Seniors will not have to buy these products solely to overcome certain hindrances or disabilities; rather, they will acquire such products because they like them. In other words, this methodology reinforces the design of senior-appropriate products that are emotionally appealing.

The methodology comprises seven dimensions subsumed under the three levels described above and noted in Figure 15.1. These shall now be briefly introduced.

Normative Level Objectives

On the normative level, our methodology has two dimensions: the salutogenetical dimension, and the target group specific dimension. In contrast to the principle of "barrier freedom," we assert that emotionally appealing technology for seniors must be tailored to their potentials rather than their disabilities. The principle of barrier freedom is based on the compensation of disabilities (Dienel & Schröder, 2000). According to this principle, senior-appropriate technology compensates for seniors' physical shortcomings. This principle is widely applied in senior housing and products for the disabled. The majority of planners and engineers working with the idea of barrier freedom for seniors still conceptualize aging as a bodily ailment. The optimal technical solution is viewed as one that best compensates for the loss of bodily functioning

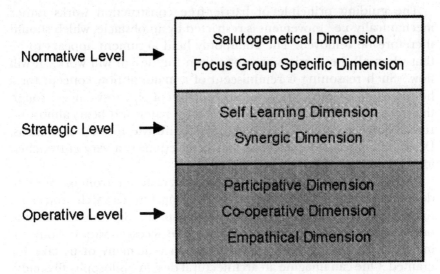

FIGURE 15.1 Objectives hierarchy determining the Sentha methodology.

associated with the aging process. This guideline is manifested in the German norms DIN 18024 (barrier-free building in public spaces) and 18025 (barrier-free building in private spaces) that cover guidelines for senior-appropriate housing. One major implication of this approach is that most products designed for seniors are stigmatized by a negative view of aging, such as portrayed in clinical geriatrics or, more generally, the negative aging stereotype.

Efforts towards barrier-free construction and barrier-free products have achieved many important goals, such as raising considerable awareness about the problems of the physically handicapped and also the elderly, among architects, product developers, and society at large. Hence, one can appreciate and endorse the principle of barrier freedom. However, this limited view does not fully encourage novel products and services.

Several existing models of barrier freedom make senior housing look dangerously similar to long-term care settings. The apartments are small, ergonomically sound, and easy to maintain and to use. Producers of domestic appliances hesitate with good reason before adopting barrier freedom as a guiding principle. However, living alone, lack of contact with the outside world, and anxiety are as important, if not more important, factors in statistics about falls than traditional examples of inappropriate doorsteps or other physical obstacles that could be removed by barrier-free construction.

The guiding principle of barrier-free construction works rather mechanically, i.e., movement is restricted by an obstacle, which should therefore be removed. The commonly held argument appears to be that when all the barriers are gone then the design will work, "it will flow." Such reasoning is reminiscent of a material flow concept for a hospital, or flow mechanics for the reduction of pipe resistance through the proper dimensions of pipes in heating systems. It bears almost no resemblance to models for an attractive lifestyle for senior citizens. Despite its obvious limitations, barrier freedom is a very entrenched idea in senior design.

One could choose guiding principles very different from barrier free design, especially in the field of senior housing. Our research project has focused on the idea of "contrasts in living space." Seniors not working outside the home or limited in mobility lose access to various contrasting spaces for living, work, and recreation that many of us take for granted. One can imagine an architectural design philosophy that cultivates contrasts in living spaces to increase quality of life, rather than focusing on the removal of all obstacles in an area. Contrasts also support attention to the environment and promote alertness toward one's physical or natural surroundings.

One well-known approach to overcome the stigmatizing aura of senior-appropriate technology is the "design-for-all" principle (universal design). We also challenge this principle and claim that a target-group specific approach is more fruitful—especially in Germany, which has a tradition of niche-oriented manufacturing. The design-for-all principle is based on an attempt to free senior-appropriate technology from an image created by its market position in special marketing channels for the disabled. Senior-appropriate technology is viewed as some sort of a medical solution to remedy a weakness or disability, and therefore it is treated as technology for a fringe group—a fringe group nobody wants to identify with since it is stigmatized as physically weak, aesthetically unattractive, and technologically uneducated. Hence, the design-for-all principle attempts to create technology that is attractive to both younger and elderly people. It is based on the idea that product design weaknesses affect all ages; the difference being that these problems are often more prevalent in the elderly.

The design-for-all principle, as we assess it, is inappropriate for the design of senior-appropriate technology. Rather, we should proactively perceive senior-appropriate technology as target group specific technology. First, we think the design-for-all principle emphasizes the stigmatizing character of senior-appropriate technology: the assumption that senior-appropriateness has to be camouflaged implicitly underlines its negative image. Secondly, we believe that the image of seniors has significantly changed over time: seniors are no longer seen only as a fringe group that is poor, technologically illiterate, and struggling with various physical disabilities. Rather, seniors become a target group that is wealthy and demands a certain high level in terms of quality of life. Therefore, seniors should be seen as a growingly affluent market segment that justifies the development of appropriate products and technology. Technology may clearly be declared as senior-appropriate; still, it has to become more attractive in order to turn its image from a fringe group technology to a target group technology. This is what we mean by emotionally appealing senior-appropriate technology. We also claim that this approach is especially fruitful in Germany since this country has been traditionally a stronghold of manufacturing and design for small groups. Germany has a long tradition of small workshops and niche manufacturing that allows customers and designers to work more closely to create new tailored products, for example, automobiles and household appliances.

STRATEGIC LEVEL OBJECTIVES

The strategic level comprises two dimensions: the self-learning dimension and the synergetic dimension. Senior-appropriate technology must be self-learning, that is, senior-appropriate technology must change, "grow" and evolve with the demands of its specific user group. Seniors, after all, are not a group characterized by somatic deficits; rather, they are characterized by potentials and preferences that may or may not change with increasing limitations in physical agility. The synergetic dimension, therefore, asks for senior-appropriate technology that meets the needs of seniors and, at the same time, is able to adjust to increasing limitations in a senior's life. For instance, imagine a senior who takes great pleasure in extensive daily bathing. She would demand a very comfortable bathtub; at the same time, she would like a bathtub that can be entered safely and effortlessly. A senior-appropriate bathtub, hence, would be a comfortable bathtub whose design is not solely determined by facilities to lift the user over the edge; rather, a senior-appropriate bathtub would be a traditional bathtub that also offers an option to be entered without having to step over a barrier or lower one's body. This is what we mean by self-learning: instead of designing a product with a certain disability to overcome in mind, products should be designed to meet a senior's preferences and at the same time they should offer the possibility to adjust to potential disabilities. This is the evolution or self-learning dimension of our methodology: technology should be designed to fulfill its core function and be able to adjust to various changing "typical" conditions and circumstances.

In order to realize the beliefs underlying these two dimensions, senior-appropriate technology must be "synergetic," e.g., a technology that cooperates with, and creates added value with, other kinds of technologies. The benefits of combining various components of synergetic technologies must be greater than the sum of each component's single benefits. Imagine again the senior that enjoys his daily bath. He would feel much more comfortable if he knew that there was a device that would call for help in case of an emergency such as a sudden fall. Of course, such a device would be developed to compensate for the disability of getting help in case of an emergency—a condition that may apply to younger people, too. However, such a device would be designed to support other products that enhance a senior's quality of life. In turn, the products should be designed to incorporate support functions. Technology is not defined as senior-appropriate due to its core function, but rather due to its adaptiveness towards additional functions. This is the synergetic dimension of senior-appropriate product development. The core function of these products remains the same—namely, to meet a senior's potential and preferences.

In summary, on the strategic level, senior-appropriate technology should take two dimensions into account. First, it should be self-learning—easily adjusting to decreasing physical agility. Secondly, it should be synergetic—easily combined with other technologies in order to adjust to decreasing physical agility.

OPERATIONAL LEVEL OBJECTIVES

For the process by which senior-appropriate products should be developed, the previous four dimensions have three major implications at the operational level: the participative dimension, the cooperative dimension, and the empathic dimension.

By participative dimension we mean that senior-appropriate technology development processes should take various perspectives into account as products are designed. We distinguish between two kinds of participation: internal participation and external participation.

- *Internal participation* encourages a multidisciplinary approach: various disciplines must be taken into account. To develop new senior-appropriate technologies, for instance, it is not sufficient to consult only construction engineers. Ergonomics experts and psychologists for example, could help designers to better understand how people might utilize new technologies. Multidisciplinarity ensures that a broad variety of scientific knowledge is considered in design and production.
- *External participation* involves engaging various societal stakeholders. For senior-appropriate products this would include seniors as well as other partners from the manufacturing industry. External participation ensures consideration of a broad variety of societal knowledge in order to develop promising products.

The participative dimension emphasizes the need to thoroughly explore numerous sources of relevant information. This ensures that products are designed to fit the exact context they are made for—in other words: the products match conditions that are more complex than just a certain, monosyndromal physical disability.

The cooperative dimension builds upon the participative approach. The whole team involved with product concept development is now assembled in a way that involves everybody in moving the product closer to market. Whereas participation relies on integrating various fields of knowledge, cooperation aims to actually integrate the knowledge and experience of various actors representing various sundry fields. Cooperation is much more flexible since it fits the process to the actors. This dimension is based on the idea that lay developers can contribute constructive ideas for senior-appropriate products. Hence, cooperation means supporting nonexpert developers with all necessary resources to generate new ideas. We believe that a major hindrance for the development of good emotional technology stems from the fact that product-relevant ideas are almost exclusively generated by experts who often have a very specific biased view, which limits the potential variety of ideas generated for senior-appropriate products. By including more actors, the cooperative dimension overcomes this limitation.

In order to develop new concepts for senior-appropriate products it might not be sufficient to explore the explicit needs of seniors. After all, seniors, like all consumers, may themselves have difficulty formulating and identifying their specific preferences. Scrutinizing seniors' behaviors provides crucial information for the design of emotional technology. This concept is often referred to as empathic scrutiny; an empathic scrutinizer would explore the conditions of a certain target group and would try to obtain information on objectives, preferences, and fears. Product developers must immerse themselves in the everyday life or "Lebenswelt" of the user group for which new products will be designed.

These three operational dimensions of senior-appropriate technologies are, of course, not mutually exclusive. Rather, an optimal product development process should synthesize the salient and useful features of all dimensions. The major idea is to find objectives on each detailed level; the normative level, the strategic level, and the operational level. These dimensions must be considered before the development process is launched.

PRODUCT DEVELOPMENT—A BRIEF OVERVIEW

When we discuss product development, we refer to the ideas developed since the 1970s by Pahl and Beitz (1997). These comprise various approaches to product development in capitalist countries categorized by objectives of product characteristics. In the 1970s, product development was driven primarily by production process limitations. Whether the products would fit certain (societal) needs was deemed less relevant. Subsequently, it became clear that successful products must meet a broader scope of objectives; for example Pahl and Beitz proposed environmentally friendly, cost-effective, modular, and easy dismantling as potential new objectives. All of the newer approaches aim to integrate societal or economic needs into the production process.

Another important related approach is conveyed in the term "participative product development" where influence, interaction, and information exchange are the most important aspects (Bullinger, 1993; Held, 1998). Influence is the key word here because participative product development basically involves designing products that meet the needs of a large set of stakeholders.

Participative product development involves two concerns at the hands-on level. It is about participative planning within a certain organization. Employees should participate through creative means of organizing work and alternative forms of human resource management (Klein, Frieling, & Ferenszkiewicz, 1989). The industry can learn from research and vice versa. The participation of potential users throughout the development of technical products is a sine qua non. Prospective users can influence product development during the whole process for products that closely fit the needs of the potential users. In this context, Raabe (1993) notes that actual product development often deviates significantly from this idea: (a) users frequently play a rather reactive (as opposed to generative) role in designing products since they are not invited to participate early in the process; (b) the competence of users is often assumed to be negligible; (c) research into markets for technologies is often of an evaluating and quantifying nature, which leaves little space for timely interaction between producers and customers. Raabe believes that wider participation by users would provide a more thorough way of thinking about marketing. Hence, developing new forms of communication between customers and product developers deserves major attention.

Obviously, it is not only in the area of senior product development that new techniques of collecting client information are being established. From videotaping shopping decision making in malls, to target groups, and tracking of Internet visits through cookies, market researchers are using increasingly inventive (and invasive) ways to get close to potential clients to understand and ultimately influence their behavior.

APPLICATION OF THE METHODOLOGY—"EVERYDAY TECHNOLOGY FOR SENIOR HOUSEHOLDS" (SENTHA)

We have described the foundations of a new comprehensive approach that enables product developers to design better assistive technology for seniors. In this section, we now describe a specific example of an application of the model.

The German research group "Everyday Technology for Senior Households" (Sentha) integrates the activities of seven institutes based at three universities and two private nonprofit research institutions, and is coordinated by the Center for Technology and Society at Berlin University of Technology. Sentha is a highly interdisciplinary research group integrating a vast variety of disciplines ranging from social science to engineering. Senior citizens and industry advisory panels also participate in the project. Sentha, therefore, is the major think tank for senior-oriented technology in Germany.

Sentha's objectives are twofold. First, it aims at developing new products and services for a new generation of seniors. As noted earlier, people in modern industrial societies have gained a new stage of life on a broad basis. This is the age after retirement, previously called "the fourth age" (Baltes & Mayer, 1999). People representing this new stage have their own approach to life—not quite young anymore, but vital, autonomous, and largely independent; they take great pleasure in life. This new and unique status is based on improved economic security for many, but not all, in old age. Sentha seeks to encourage the development of products that enhance this new quality of life. Technology—according to the Sentha model—is "a friend of old age." Second, Sentha uses technologies for senior citizens as examples to test and develop new participatory approaches to technological design, thus contributing to interdisciplinary product development. These approaches can be formulated as one model of product development that encourages the design of emotional technology, while building upon current core principles of product development.

Sentha has developed numerous product ideas and concepts in cooperation with seniors. Seniors have tested new products and services in Sentha's ergonomic development lab, the Learning Home, a simulation environment and laboratory for product design. Among its major aims are realization, demonstration, testing, and evaluation of product concepts. For instance, networks, control tools, and sensors as well as user interfaces and speech processing tools are already installed in the Learning Home. Researchers can join, discuss, and present ideas, or invite seniors to discuss ideas with them. It is a physical space in which cooperation can take place.

The Learning Home also functions serendipitously as what is called "a boundary object" (Star, 1989; Star & Griesemer, 1989) in the sociology of science. Boundary objects are objects that facilitate the translation among different social worlds. They have to be "both plastic enough to adapt to local needs and constraints of the several parties employing them, yet robust enough to maintain a common identity across sites" (Star, 1989, p. 46). Two results are important in this regard:

1. A major aspect enhancing the quality of a cooperation is cohabitation (Dienel & Schröder, 2000), a common space where cooperating partners work and communicate. In Sentha, cohabitation is realized since the Learning Home creates a locus for face-to-face meetings and cooperative experiments for organizations that are otherwise geographically dispersed.

2. The new collaborations made possible by the Learning Home also made it necessary to jointly think about concepts, ideas, and methods for the best use of the facility. The Learning Home proved to

be a conceptual focal point facilitating joint research and development efforts consistent with the Sentha methodology described earlier in this chapter.

The Learning Home reinforces cooperation among heterogeneous partners both physically and conceptually. It is similar to the research facility "Living Lab" at the British Columbia Institute of Technology (BCIT) in Vancouver described in the chapter by Watzke.

Both these facilities allow for researchers to observe and videotape seniors as they use products. The question then becomes how to use these tools in a way where seniors are not just observed objects but are active participants in the design and execution of the experiments. Modern technologies such as wearable computers that monitor body functions, global positioning systems that can trace movements, and smart cards that track every purchase can make seniors lives more convenient but also present new challenges to their autonomy. Constructing innovative methods of product design and testing also requires us to be conscious of new risks to active participation.

Sentha's project ideas are the integrated knowledge of all participating institutes—thus, they are interdisciplinary. Efficient and effective cooperation did not, at first, come easily but a certain procedure emerged which was very helpful and promising for further interdisciplinary work. Specifically we found that the process of generating product concepts should include the following steps:

1. *The Creativity Phase.* Throughout this phase, various creativity techniques are applied to generate a broad variety of product ideas. Each discipline may generate its own ideas; this ensures that the cooperative dimension is properly considered. Product ideas are tested against the criteria on the strategic level; that is, ideas that are explored more closely must show *self-learning* and *synergetic* potential.

2. *The Development Phase.* Throughout this phase, various ideas that passed the test against the strategic criteria are elaborated more fully. The ideas are validated by various disciplines so that each discipline gets input from others on how to proceed with the idea, (internal participative dimension) and the senior advisory panel contributes to the elaboration (external participative dimension). At the conclusion of this phase, each product idea is represented in a detailed written description and in a physical model.

3. *The Evaluation Phase.* Throughout this phase, product ideas are evaluated for their strengths and weaknesses. Based on the detailed elaboration, the idea is tested against the opinions of a significant number of seniors. At the end of this phase, it is decided which ideas will be abandoned and which ideas will be developed into prototypes.

4. *The Improvement Phase.* The previous steps are referred to as a product development cycle. Based on experiences gained throughout one particular circle, the cycle is often repeated. Certain methods might have proven to be unsuitable while others might be highly promising.

CONCLUSION, FURTHER RESEARCH, AND OUTLOOK

Further research has still to be conducted to refine and validate this model. Whereas some dimensions such as the participative and the cooperative dimension can be easily translated into practical steps, others such as the empathic dimension remain to be fully explored. Whereas our methodology is tailored to the specific context of assistive technology, we propose that it can also be generalized to a generic methodology allowing for better, that is, more emotional, product development. We summarize with a review of steps necessary to properly evaluate our methodology and develop it into a fully elaborated tool.

First, new target groups must be defined. In order to find the information necessary to strengthen our framework, various contexts have to be explored. One way of systematically thinking about such contexts is to consider potential target groups. Such groups could be subgroups of seniors (that is intellectual seniors, practical seniors, or elderly foreigners with limited capabilities with the native language) or could be completely different target groups.

Second, new product sectors must be identified. After all, the methodology is about developing products. In order to do so, various product sectors such as mobile communication or rehabilitation technologies must be examined. We assume that our methodology will vary with the products we design.

Third, the methodology must be tested in an entrepreneurial context and integrated with existing marketing principles and systems. In order to unfold its whole potential, the methodology must work in a commercial environment. After all, businesses rather than research groups develop products. Hence, the methodology must be practical enough to be applied quickly and easily. This will be a major task for further research.

Finally, our methodology focuses on the soft aspects of products—aspects that relate to such vague issues as emotional preferences. The way people perceive technology becomes as important as the objective properties of that technology. Our methodology provides a way to take these emotional aspects of technology assessment into account in the product development process.

ACKNOWLEDGMENTS

Hans Liudger Dienel is Acting Director, Alexander Peine is Research Fellow, and Heather Cameron is SSHRC Post Doctoral Fellow, of the Centre for Technology and Society, Technical University of Berlin, Germany.

REFERENCES

Baltes, P. B., & Mayer, K. U. (Eds.) (1999). *The Berlin ageing study: Ageing from 70 to 100.* New York: Cambridge University Press.

Bullinger, H.-J. (Ed.) (1993). *Kundenorientierte Produktion. Wettberwerbsfaktor Arbeitsorganisation.* Stuttgart: IAO

Dienel, H.-L., & Schröder, C. (2000). Kohabitation und multidisziplinäre Forschung. Innovation durch Perspektivenvergleich. In H. -J. Harloff, et al. (Eds.): *Wohnen und Nachhaltigkeit: Interdisziplinäre Forschung vor der Haustür.* Berlin: Berlin Institute of Technology Press.

Goleman, D. (1997). *Emotional intelligence:Why it can matter more than IQ.* New York: Bantam Books.

Held, J. P. (1998). *Partizipative Ergonomie: Die Prozessgestaltung zur Beteiligung Betroffener an ergonomischen Gestaltungsaufgaben.* Zürich: Diss.

Keeney, R. L. (1992). *Value-focused thinking: A path to creative decision making.* Cambridge: Harvard University Press.

Klein, H., Frieling, E., & Ferenszkiewicz, D. (1989). *Veränderungsperspektiven im Konstruktionsbereich. Erfahrungen mit partizipativer Organisations- und Personalentwicklung.* Düsseldorf: VDI.

Olbrich, E. (1999). Menschengerechte Produktgestaltung: Schnittstelle zwischen der Person und ihrer Umwelt. In H.-L. Dienel, Foerster, C., Hentschel, B., Zorn, C., & Blanckenburg, C. (Eds.) (1999). Technik, Freundin des Alters: Vergangenheit und Zukunft spАᵒter Freiheiten. Stuttgart: Steiner.

Pahl, G., & Beitz, W. (1997). *Konstruktionslehre, Methode und Anwendung, 4th ed.* Berlin: Springer Publishing.

Quade, E. S. (1985). Objectives, constraints and alternatives. In H. J. Miser & E. S. Quade (Eds.), *Handbook of systems analysis: Overview of uses, procedures, applications and practice*, Volume 1. Chichester: Wiley.

Raabe, T. (1993). *Konsumentenbeteiligung an der Produktinnovation*. Frankfurt: Main.

Selle, K. (1996*). Planung und Kommunikation*. Heidelberg: Bauverlag.

Star, S. L. (1989). The Structure of Ill-Structured Solutions: Boundary Objects and Heterogeneous Distributed Problem Solving. In L. Gasser & M. N. Huhns (Eds.), *Distributed Intelligence*. London: Pitman.

Star, S. L., & Griesemer, J. R. (1989). Institutional ecology, 'translations' and boundary objects: Amateurs and professionals in Berkeley's Museum of Vertebrate Zoology, 1907–39. *Social Studies of Science, 19*, 387–420.

Section E

Cautions, Integration, and Synthesis

16

Ethical Realities: The Old, the New, and the Virtual

Gari Lesnoff-Caravaglia

Dimensions of time have commonly followed a forward movement based principally on the observations of physical changes in the environment, the cycles of seasons, and alterations in human development. Such changes were viewed as given and the result of dictates of external forces of either mystical or physical origin. The inalterability of such changes provided structure for human knowledge, understanding, and belief. This view was held by major philosophers, including Kant. The spatial location of the individual within time was viewed as delimited in physical duration by birth and death (Beckman, 1998).

The increasing exposure to speed within time coupled with the indifference to spatial location, however, has catapulted human experience into an ambiguous and formless confusion. The known has become the unknown; the familiar, strange, and the dream, reality. The person as physical entity has become insignificant. The realm of knowledge is without mooring and captained by special interests. Fiction has supplanted fact, which is prey to the hustling of political interests, special interests, and the entertainment industry. Individual thought unhesitatingly reflects a common, blotter-like uniformity (Virilio, 2000).

Early in the twentieth century, the German philosopher Martin Heidegger delineated the form of very real ethical and spiritual crises that a world dominated by technology and scientific formulations would inspire. Following World War I, there was a strong protest against the secure cultural world of the older generation and the leveling of all traditional forms of life by industrial society to an increasing uniformity (Gadamer, 1976). The inevitable linkage between economic, political, and social power engendered by technology was seen as potentially altering the basis of human reference to persons and the environment. There was the danger of regarding persons and the natural world as solely instruments for profit and gain. Human thought would be subsumed to meet industrialization's needs, to the detriment of persons, cultures, and the natural world (Heidegger, 1977; Sheehan, 1981; Tipler, 1994).

In the contemporary view, the entire universe is perceived in terms of its value for the promotion and exercise of human power. The value of objects or persons lies in their utility. The universe itself is regarded as an objective, mathematically quantifiable field of energy open to investigation. Only that which can be examined in exact formulations by science is considered to be real. All else is assumed to be based on superstition. For philosophers such as Heidegger, the essence of technology is that reality is viewed as calculable, rational (mathematical), and thus controllable (Sheehan, 1981). This view of reality, however, has the subtle power of engulfing human beings so that the objective view of the universe begins inexorably to become identified with human beings as well. Calculative thinking predominates at the expense of ethical and moral reasoning. The danger of seeing the world as a manipulable object is to lose sight of the relationship between the universe and human beings and can result in a more barren wasteland than the effects of atomic weaponry. Current ecological concerns are mirrored in this possibility.

Technological innovation has inevitably and irretrievably altered the course of human lives. It continues to evoke strong positive and negative reactions. The introduction of a new technology presents the possibility of several unforeseen consequences. The potential for accident or malfunction is inherent in the invention. For example, the development of the ship carried with it the potential for shipwrecks. The invention of the railway meant, perforce, the invention of the railway disaster. The airplane brought the air crash in its wake, while the automobile introduced the automobile accident. Primary emphasis has been placed on the invention itself without foreseeing the potential malfunction or accident that arises as an inevitable consequence. Some disasters, such as nuclear accidents, can have global effects, such as the destruction of the entire world. Geography thus becomes insignificant (Virilio, 2000).

Increases in life expectancy to the age of 125 and beyond can also be conceptualized in this manner. The effects of such life extension upon individuals and society have yet to be fully assessed. There may well be future references to the "accident" of old age.

THE HUMAN ENTERPRISE

The early introduction of technology was viewed with enthusiasm as it was first applied to help conquer the natural environment. The ability to dominate the natural world was viewed as unlimited progress. The pervasive view that inspires the creation and utilization of technology can also be seen as resulting in humans falling under the influence of the machines they have created. While not ignoring the benefits of many of the current technologies, the nature of the thinking that is initiated by their very presence has resulted in such domination. In short, technology has inevitably provided systems which ultimately control human behavior.

The ongoing ecological crisis, the dangers of technological weaponry, the growing sense of helplessness felt by those who are victimized by gigantic corporations and bureaucracies all contribute to the growing awareness that individuals have little control over their fates (Gilleard & Higgs, 2000). The heaven on earth promised by the introduction of technologies appears not to have been fulfilled. There is an increasing uneasiness that something has gone awry. Technology rather than enhancing the role of the individual has effectively diminished it. Furthermore, when people are viewed as *capital,* the elderly become expendable. When people must travel miles from their concrete enclaves before they can see a tree, the divorce of humans and the natural universe is conclusive.

The human enterprise is largely based upon choice and self-realization. The continual and growing presence of technology has subtly and persistently both enlarged and diminished human freedom. Such waxing and waning of human possibilities has extended to the alteration of the functioning of the human organism through expediencies such as the transplanting of body parts to the cessation of participation in one's own demise (Lesnoff-Caravaglia, 1999).

Conversely, technology has led to increased sensitivity to the humanitarian aspects of science and technology in terms of their responsibilities to human existence and the environment. The freedom of continued life through radical medical interventions continues apace. Alteration of the environment is also conducive to life enhancement and increased life expectation with robotic capabilities assuming the role of the extension of self.

The word "robot" was invented in 1920 by the Bohemian writer Karel Capek. In Czech the word "robota" signifies work. However, it was principally following World War II with the advent of electronics that the myth of the robot emerged. Numerous films and books described the science fiction world where humans would no longer need to exert themselves, as the most mundane tasks of life would be taken over by robots (Lesnoff-Caravaglia, 2001).

Perhaps the most visionary writers of that period, Isaac Asimov, predicted that by the year 2000 robots might rebel against humans, flaunting slogans based on the statement by Descartes: *Cogito, ergo sum* (I think, therefore, I am). The prediction has not been realized, although robots are prevalent in settings such as industry and medicine. Unfortunately, while computerized robots have revolutionized these fields, the effects upon the lives of average citizens have not been as telling. The myth of the robot that does the housecleaning and prepares the meals has been perpetuated for some thirty years, with few concrete results.

Today, machines are still simple creations, requiring the parental care and protective nurturing of any newborn, hardly worthy of the word "intelligent." They will, however, mature into something transcending everything currently known and may well be viewed as human descendants, while the humans of today gradually disappear (Moravec, 1988).

The industrial revolution of several centuries ago initiated the artificial substitution for human body functions such as lifting and transporting. The computational power of mechanical devices has risen a thousand times every twenty years since then. Soon, virtually no essential human function, physical or mental, will lack an artificial counterpart. This convergence of cultural developments will result in the intelligent robot, a machine that can think and act as a human, however inhuman it may be in physical or mental detail. Such machines could carry on the cultural evolution, including their own construction and increasingly rapid self-improvement, without human presence or the benefit of human genes. The evolutionary process will have moved on to a new competitor or form (Moravec, 1988). The culture can then evolve independently of human biology and its limitations, passing directly from generation to generation of ever more capable intelligent machinery.

The future association between humans and machines may well be in the form of a partnership. In time, the relationship may devolve to a more symbiotic one with less evident boundary between the human and mechanical partner. Some of this is already manifest in the utilization of artificial organs and other body parts, often superior to the original. There is the potential to replace everything in the form of a new body, a specially designed robot body.

The additional element of the proper "fit" of human choice within the scope of constant and unremitting change poses significant dilemmas regarding human freedom. Society's acceptance of particular technologies can place limitations on personal choice or alter the framework from which choice is perceived. Such alterations can hamper the individual's self-determination and ability to maintain a personal identity, incursions due to debility, frailty, and age notwithstanding (Lesnoff-Caravaglia, 1988).

AGING AND THE ERA OF TECHNOLOGY

The reciprocal relationship between technology and aging provides both challenges and opportunities. The societal effects of technological change and the aging of the population are likely to be felt in various ways: health status, living environments, and work. The creation, dissemination and use of technology involves not only a mastery of sciences and engineering tools and concepts, but the ability to cope with a difficult set of ethical and economic issues and choices.

The unprecedented demographic and technological changes have brought to the forefront the issues of the quality of life and the nature of the life that is to be continued. New production and workplace technologies alter the nature of labor and the requisites of the work force. The prevalence of chronic illnesses and attendant functional impairments among nonagenarians and centenarians will rise as the proportion of people in these age categories increases, resulting in significant changes in family structure and living arrangements.

The Swiss architect LeCorbusier once stated that a home is a machine for living in. That insight has become more meaningful than ever with the advent of new prospects such as the Smart House.

HUMAN EXPERIENCE WITHIN
EXTRAORDINARY FRAMEWORKS

When the railroad and the automobile first came upon the scene, those who so desired still had the option to travel by various means, including horseback. This option no longer exists. A businessman cannot acquire a computer just because he likes progress. The computer implies networks; it brings a whole system with it. The technical system has now become strongly integrated within offices, means of production, and personnel. Its proper use helps maintain order within society. The incorporation of nuclear energy or genetic engineering follows the same pattern; their proper or improper use challenges philosophical concepts and ethical positions (Ellul, 1990).

Descartes (1960) may have been more than prophetic in his description of human experience as a phenomenon of the mind. He maintained that individuals never really directly perceive things; they just perceive things as happening in their minds or brains. Virtual experience has much of exactly this element. The computer has supplanted the real world, and the world is experienced intellectually, not actually.

Virilio (1997) expanded this theme when he describes a contemporary movement that is intensifying due to remote control and long-distance telepresence technologies. Their presence can result in an increasingly sedentary society composed of overequipped, able-bodied persons. Virilio further states:

> Service or servitude . . . that is the question. The old public services are in danger of being replaced by a domestic enslavement whose crowning glory would surely be home automation. Achieving a domiciliary inertia, the widespread use of techniques of environmental control will end in behavioral isolation, in intensifying the insularity . . . (p. 20).

There are real similarities between the state of reduced mobility of the well-equipped disabled person and the growing inertia of the overequipped, able-bodied person. It is the nature of the contemporary world that produces this effect. In the way that the European well-to-do developed private chapels in their home, entertainment centers figure prominently in homes throughout the industrialized world.

The inert, sedentary lifestyle characterizes much of society. Telecommunication has led to a transparent horizon that allows physical presence in one place and, at the same time, phantom participation in events on the opposite side of the world. Physical action is no longer required to alter one's life space. Drapes, lights, room temperature, doors, and appliances can be instantaneously controlled through remote control.

Escalators and elevators are preferred over stairs, and walking is reduced by the use of moving walkways. Sports are enjoyed by watching others, sitting as observers in specially developed stadiums which often include restaurants as observation points, or sitting at home in the privacy of personal entertainment centers. This observing is usually accompanied by the consumption of food and drink of high caloric content that reinforces the sedentary lifestyle through unhealthy diet practices and consequent obesity.

In office practices it is easier to send electronic mail than to post a letter or to use a messenger. The resulting abbreviated, short-hand messages and ungrammatical usage have led to the universal corruption of language and eliminated any literary pretensions of written correspondence. The language of the telegram is rapidly becoming the acceptable mode of communication.

The rapid movement of persons from one place to another across the globe is an accepted characteristic of contemporary society. "Departure" and "arrival" bear greater significance than the trip itself. People are moved from one point to another via airplanes and bullet trains in a state of passivity that borders on unconsciousness as they sleep, watch films, or daydream hurtled through space. The space intervening the "departure" and "arrival" becomes a vacuum empty of content, enjoyment, or intellectual stimulation. It is the "arrival" only that has significance. The speed of arrival of persons, messages, and television reporting is the paramount interest. The use of the remote control has the same effect in domestic environments (Virilio, 1997).

The human space is made ambiguous, and it is difficult to ascertain personal boundaries, the borders of states, provinces, or countries. The geographic terrain becomes immaterial. The amorphous world makes it difficult to distinguish one's personal space, the private from the public, and confuses the here and now with points distant. Such distancing of the self from real-time experience modifies levels of control and choice. By utilizing the remote control, the individual is convinced that he or she is in control of personal life space. This also explains the popularity and ubiquity of the cellular phone. For some persons, in fact, the extent of the control is even more limiting when the body has been subjected to internal alterations through advanced medical practices such as transplants. Having been placed in the position of being a constant recipient of technological interventions, internal as well as external, human experience is inevitably tied to a sedentary life. The end result is that the body appears to be wired to its life space (Virilio, 1997).

PERSONAL IDENTITY AND AGING

Human aging can be likened to a battle of resistance: to the physical outward appearances of age; the social stigmatization and ostracism, particularly in the case of women; the decline in power and influence; and the warding off of disease as aging advances. No one chooses to grow old, especially in a youth-oriented society. The redefinition of self is an individual project often restricted by cultural and ethical parameters. Future developments in technology may play an increasing role in shaping this definition.

In response to alterations in the physical environment, the human body experiences alterations that are in concert with environmental demands. Some such alterations are transplant procedures or the implanting of devices deep within a human body. The arrangement of the domestic environment facilitates the consolidation of the person to the "smart house." In the near future there may well be an increased fusion of the biological and the technological. It is already predicted that the majority of surgical procedures in the future will be on the order of organ transplants and the implanting of a variety of prostheses. The goal of such prostheses may include the enhancement or ameliorization of sensory functions such as vision and hearing beyond what are currently considered normal capabilities. Night vision, distance hearing, and specialized gloves for tactile discrimination are increasingly part of the technological armamentarium.

The increasing proliferation of technological changes challenges societies to understand how the changes promise to affect human life and to direct thinking toward the future. The rate of change in society today is largely the result of the ability to manipulate the world to suit particular needs. This "technologizing" of the world is in a very real sense an evolutionary process which encompasses internal as well as external changes. The effects upon future life are unclear and often lead to a sense of dismal foreboding, stress, anxiety, and depression (Lesnoff-Caravaglia, 2000).

The response of the human system to environmental conditions is exemplified by the experiences of the cosmonauts. After a few weeks in space, a cosmonaut's body begins to rebuild itself. The effect of weightlessness means that the heart no longer needs to pump blood so powerfully upwards. The veins and arteries restructure themselves to acclimatize, the muscles of the heart break down and change shape. Upon return from his final mission on the defunct space station Mir, which had lasted one year and two weeks, double the time he had planned for, Sergei Avdeyev, the Russian cosmonaut, was brought out of the capsule on a stretcher. He was too weak to walk and unable to sit up in a chair without slumping forward. It was a year before his heart repaired itself, and his body readjusted to gravity.

Avdeyev slept in a floating sleeping bag attached to the wall of one of the station's side modules. He described sleeping in a weightless environment as very comfortable once he got used to it. Any position, whether face up or down, on the right side or left side, all felt the same. One determines for oneself where is up, and then one can pretend to be sleeping lying down, with a pillow under one's head. The concept of what is the ceiling and what is the floor is all in the mind.

Such alterations in self/world perception are also mirrored in the sense of the rapid passage of time. It is exhausting to live in a world in which everything is timed to the minute or second. There is little attention paid to seasonal rhythms. The fundamental fact is that all organisms are at the height of their vigor and powers in spring and summer. In autumn and winter (until hibernation), all organisms lose their vital force (Ellul, 1990). Artificial light has made it possible to live as much at night as during the day. The basic life rhythms are ignored.

Within such changing contexts, the effort for older persons to remain self-determined is daunting. The situation can possibly be best described as "Maslow in reverse." In Maslow's pyramid, people satisfy basic needs and move up to the top or pinnacle of the pyramid to reach a personal sense of achievement in intellectual or spiritual arenas. Older persons have spent their lives striving to reach the top of the pyramid, and many achieve this task successfully. Now that they are at the top of the pyramid and are aged, they must move downward, backwards in some sense, and this is a negative progression that is not happily attempted. To move down from the top means preoccupation with psychological and biological functioning. Since such basic needs had once been mastered, there may be anger and frustration at having to attend so exclusively to meeting them, particularly when one's tolerance and ability to cope are waning. This move also constitutes a radical change in self image and those intellectual, spiritual, or professional achievements that form part of self-identity pale against the reality of negotiating a steep flight of stairs or opening a food container. For older persons, intellectual, professional, spiritual, aesthetic, and avocational growth seems to have been dismissed, disregarded, or diminished in meaning (Lesnoff-Caravaglia, 1999, 2001).

TECHNOLOGY AND THE WORLD OF THE OLDER WOMAN

Technological innovation has markedly affected where, how, why, and even when women age. The lack of "fit" between the person and the environment is particularly striking in the world of the older woman and has resulted in premature aging and the escalation of disease states. The absence of alterations in environments such as public places, dwelling, and institutions frequented by older women has circumscribed their lives and caused them to age more rapidly and to experience higher rates of illness than their chronological age alone might warrant. The ignoring of such factors is not only an indication of gender bias, but is a reflection of social apathy and the fact that linking technology to aging has become an academic exercise with few roots in reality.

The much discussed "smart house" has left no one the wiser. Older women continue to live in antiquated environments, and the much condemned "grab-bar mentality" has remained as the only signal advance. The freedom and independence to be afforded by recent technological advances has not been reflected in the home setting, in institutions providing services to older women, nor in the lifestyles of older women. Despite such advancements in technology, older women continue to live in an obsolete world.

The environment as the locus for aging largely influences why particular physiological and psychological changes are experienced with advancing age. Public and private environments that do not adequately match the needs and capabilities of older women often serve to accelerate the aging process. Inhospitable environments are responsible for the increase in stress that accompanies aging, as well as increasing the potential for accidents and reducing healthful behaviors such as meal preparation, personal hygiene, and physical activity.

Prosthetic or adaptive environments that are technologically malleable can serve to extend the capacities of aging women and to promote continued maximal functioning. Robotic and artificial intelligence in human-machine integration provides unprecedented opportunities for maximizing human functional potential. Yet, the home environment continues unchanged, and "home" becomes less sweet and more lethal as its occupants age.

Even the more spectacular biological interventions have been without an echo. Artificial or assistive insemination has radically altered reproductive possibilities for older women, even after menopause. Such advances have led some nations to consider instituting laws to prevent older women from being impregnated after reaching a certain age. One argument offered to support such legislation is that the older woman would be too old to nurture children in late life. It is interesting to note that such an argument has never been advanced when the aged parent is a male. The capacity to successfully implant a uterus is a new effort to overcome menopause and to continue female fertility indefinitely. In contrast to the discovery of Viagra, this discovery did not make headlines. In the meantime, Viagra has become a term as commonplace as Kleenex (Lesnoff-Caravaglia, 2001).

CENTANNI OR LONG LIFE

The goal of one hundred years—*centanni* (the traditional Sicilian toast)—has long been surpassed. People live as children for 15 years, as an adolescent for 5, as a young adult for 20, as middle aged for 20, and for as long as 60 as an older person. The second half of life is lived as an older person. Much of this extension of life can be attributed to the advancements in health care and medical research. Ethical dilemmas abound with respect to when, where, and how to utilize such medical interventions. They involve the deliberations of physicians, social workers, and third-party payers who become, in fact, gatekeepers in terms of health care allocation. When would a person be considered too old to be given a particular device? What is the rationale for keeping older persons alive when they suffer from irreversible brain disease or dementia? The responses to such questions become increasingly more complex as medical technology and science continue to advance and to provide alternative treatment possibilities. Technology now can control the timing and quality of individual demise.

The human body is endowed from birth with many natural defenses, including autoimmunity and redundancy of tissues, organs, and parts, enabling it to resist the changes that come with age, disease, and trauma. As human beings age, such natural defenses gradually fail and may require replacements. The growing number of medical devices and instrumentation that has characterized modern health care, along with transplants, may well substitute for loss of such natural defenses. This may also pave the way for the technological control of human bodily functions.

Technological advances in the medical-device area have had a profound impact on patient survival and improved quality of life. The benefits have been particularly notable for chronic conditions that become more prevalent with increasing age. Initially technical aids were not popular with health care professionals who resisted their introduction into patient care. This has been particularly the case in adopting new devices to facilitate patient mobility and those that alter existing routines in patient care. Since the introduction of such technologies can enhance the lives of older persons, one might well argue whether their restricted or nonuse is an infringement on the rights of older patients.

SEX AND DEMOGRAPHY

The "virtual love" permitted by the sensory feats of cybersex may well have dire consequences for human demography. The computer, in this sense, can be regarded as "a universal condom" (Virilio, 1997, p. 67). The result is a loss of tangible reality that has had its echo in high divorce rates and the growth of single-parent families. At a time when innovations are occurring in artificial fertilization and genetic engineering, with the aid of biocybernetic accoutrements using sensor-effectors distributed over the genital organs, conjugal relations between opposite sexes have been short-circuited and coitus interrupted. Tactile telepresence (touching at a distance) allows partners in virtual love to engage in a cybernetic process in which the operator console is no longer satisfied just to synthesize images or sound, it can also orchestrate sexual sensations. If the virtual pleasure of sexual telepresence were eventually to outstrip the real pleasure of embodied love, those societies left to ensure the continuation of the human race will be those that are underdeveloped and, worse, media-deprived (Virilio, 1997). Boundaries between biology and technology, humans and machines, are being effaced one by one.

In regard to older individuals, Viagra for some older men has meant continued participation in sexual activity. For older women, the possibility of artificial insemination and uterus transplants hold promise for continued procreativity even in advanced years. The drop in fertility rates among younger persons can potentially in the future be balanced by older families resulting from sexually active and fertile older couples.

In another context, sexuality can become truly age irrelevant through available expediencies such as the Internet. Persons can adopt whatever age they please and can assume attributes that will make them sexually desirable. A woman of 70 can portray herself as being 35, or can imagine herself in the guise of a much younger version of herself, thus reliving her past in the present. Cosmetic surgery also allows for such incursions into the past by permitting persons the opportunity to turn back the years through reframing or reshaping the body. Technology thus can permit choice as to when and how one ages.

THE "BAD" REPUTATION OF MACHINES

The aesthetic qualities of machines have long been maligned. "People bored with the general blatancy of machine-made 'progress' have had a dislike of machines. The association of machines with ugliness or discomfort or pandemonium is very strong" (Pound, 1996, p. 59). Contemporary sculpture and architecture have incorporated aspects of the clean utilitarian profiles of machines. The beauty and simplicity of the machine in terms of function and motion has been undervalued until recently.

Machines are not intrinsically bad. In fact, the problem lies with the public and persons who use machines but do not understand them. Machines can be friends and helpers to human beings who are, themselves, imprecise machines. The body itself is a sort of microcosm of the machine. The arms are levers, the lungs bellows, the eyes lenses, the heart a pump, the fist a hammer, and the nerves a telegraph system connected with a central station. On the whole, however, the mechanical instruments were invented before the physiological functions were accurately described (Mori, 1981).

In addition, a drafting machine can draw a hundred or more perfect circles all the same size, but a human has difficulty in drawing even one. People cannot use gases or liquids with their hands, but machines can handle them through the use of pipes and pumps. Repetitive or odious tasks can be performed better by machines. Machines, however, are incapable of analyzing the nature of a complicated problem or grasping the total meaning of a particular line of reasoning (Mori, 1981). Those who argue the obsolescence of humankind overlook the essential difference between humans and machines: A machine has neither instinct nor will and cannot change the course of its action even in the presence of danger.

Ethical dilemmas do arise in the cohabitation of humans with machines. It is almost unavoidable that the human environment and the humans living within that space undergo change. Humans develop attitudes and behaviors that did not exist prior to the mechanical age. The nature of the combination of technologized human beings and the machines can be viewed as positive or negative, but it is certain that the mix will continue to form and reform itself over time. Technology and aging are very similar in one respect—they both have an onward or forward movement. There is no going back. Once a technology is invented and it proves to be useful, it is changed only to become even more complex and does not disappear. Aging also moves forward in an inexorable fashion. In this sense, technology and aging are both structured by time.

THE GERONTOCRACY

It may well occur that societal power in the future will reside in the elderly. It is possible that the day of Plato's philosopher king has arrived.

> Should power reside in age, one might well find in vogue the trembling hand and shuffling gait, spectacles and hearing aid. The young feigning sensory loss and graying the hair or attempting its removal in an effort to appear venerable.
>
> If the pace to be emulated is slow and measured, then the impatience and haste of youth is put to shame. When caution is preferred over imprudence, and deliberate action over trial and error, then youth is a lament and old age a herald.
>
> When age is feared—not because of the proximity of death, but as the centrifugal force of life—then idolatry of youth will fade as will smoked glass and candlelight as fitting accoutrements for women of age. (Lesnoff-Caravaglia, 1984, p. 9)

ACKNOWLEDGMENTS

Gari Lesnoff-Caravaglia is Professor, School of Health Sciences, Ohio University, Athens, Ohio.

REFERENCES

Beckman, J. (Ed.) (1998). *The virtual dimension.* New York: Princeton Architectural Press.

Descartes, R. (1960). *Discourse on method and meditations: Rules for the direction of the mind.* Indianapolis, IN: Bobbs-Merrill.

Ellul, J. (1990). *The technological bluff.* Grand Rapids, MI: W. B. Eerdmans.

Gadamer, H. (1976). *Philosophical hermeneutics.* (D. Linge, Translation). Berkeley, CA: University. of California Press.

Gilleard, C., & Higgs, P. (2000). *Cultures of aging. Self, citizen and the body.* Harlow, England: Prentice-Hall.

Heidegger, M. (1977). *The question concerning technology and other essays.* (W. Lovitt, Translation). New York: Garland Publishers., Inc.

Lesnoff-Caravaglia, G. (Ed.) (1984). *The world of the older woman.* New York: Human Sciences Press.

Lesnoff-Caravaglia, G. (1988). Aging in a technological society. In G. Lesnoff-Caravaglia (Ed.), *Aging in a technological society.* New York: Human Sciences Press.

Lesnoff-Caravaglia, G. (1999). Ethical issues in a high-tech society. In T. F. Johnson (Ed.), *Handbook on ethical issues in aging.* Westport, CT: Greenwood Press.

Lesnoff-Caravaglia, G. (2000). *Health aspects of aging. The experience of growing old.* Springfield, IL: C. C. Thomas.

Lesnoff-Caravaglia, G. (Ed.) (2001). *Aging and public health: Technology and demography: Parallel evolutions.* Springfield, IL: C. C. Thomas.

Moravec, H. (1988). *Mind children: The future of robot and human intelligence.* Cambridge, MA: Harvard University Press.

Mori, M. (1981). *The Buddha in the robot.* (C. S. Terry, Translation). Tokyo: Kosei Publishing Co.

Pound, E. (1996). *Machine art & other writings.* Durham, NC: Duke University Press.

Sheehan, T. (Ed.) (1981). *Heidegger: The man and the thinker.* Chicago: Precedent Publishing, Inc.

Tipler, F. (1994). *The physics of immortality.* New York: Doubleday.

Virilio, P. (1997). *Open sky.* New York: Verso.

Virilio, P. (2000). *Polar inertia.* (P. Camiller, Translation). Thousand Oaks, CA: Sage.

Epilogue:
Applications to Aging Are Helping Human Factors and Ergonomics To Grow Up Right

James L. Fozard

The applications of human factors and ergonomics to the challenges and opportunities of aging contribute both to an improved quality of life for older persons and to the quality of transactional person/environment models frequently used in gerontology. This epilogue develops these two themes with an emphasis on the second.

WORK ON AGING INCLUDES BOTH COMPONENTS OF ERGONOMICS AND HUMAN FACTORS

The first definition of human factors and ergonomics I learned was provided by Dr. Alphonse Chapanis in a lecture given when I was a graduate student and research assistant at San Diego State University helping prepare the Joint Armed Services Annotated Bibliography of Human Factors in Design (Chapanis & McCollom, 1956). His definition, "engineering for human use," had nothing to do with aging. The definition emphasized that when employing a tool to accomplish a task, the person and the device should be considered together as a person/environment or man/machine system. Engineering for human use requires analysis of system performance in order to "optimize it" by proper assignment of system functions to man or machine.

OPTIMIZING USER INTERFACES IN EXISTING SYSTEMS

"Optimizing system performance" acquires various operational meanings depending on the application. One class of operational definitions involves user interface improvements of existing systems, usually by optimizing the configuration of the machine's displays and controls relative to the limitations of the human user. The majority of success stories in human factors are based on this approach, including most of the material in the present volume. Examples include chapters in section C, (Hammel & Sabata) and section D (Ujimoto; Dienel, Cameron, & Peine; Watzke). The chapters describe advances in the use of assistive technology for carrying out everyday household and work tasks. Other chapters in section D also reflect this approach, especially the chapters by Tran, and by Rebok and Keyl. Age-related declines in cognitive and perceptual functioning that require special consideration in design are discussed in section A (Scialfa, Ho, & LaBerge; Mayhorn, Rogers & Fisk), and in section B (Benbow; Smyth & Kwon; Morrell, Mayhorn, & Echt). These chapters consider both system redesign and training of older users as compensatory interventions for age-related functional limitations.

OPTIMAL ASSIGNMENT OF SYSTEM
FUNCTION TO MAN OR MACHINE

The second class of operational definitions of "engineering for human use" is closer to the original design process of the system—the proper initial assignment of system functions to man or machine. In application, the system analysis attempts to insure that the technology makes the best use of the human and machine components' system capacities.

My first job in ergonomics used this approach. I worked with the late Robert Lockard on a project to replace the manually operated controls of the machines used to move the motion picture cameras that recorded the trajectories of missiles (Lockard & Fozard, 1956). Further attempts to improve either the optical display or the gain-adjustable manual tracking controls were not sufficient to meet task requirements. We developed and evaluated the idea of obtaining a signal from eye movements made by the operator while tracking the missile to drive the movements of the tracking system. Contemporary applications based on this approach include the use of individually adapted voice controls for computers, substitution of light pen pointers for mouse and keyboards, and control systems based on "smart," self-adapting software.

The optimal assignment of system function to humans has been reflected in many important types of applications for aging users. Population stereotypes or user expectations about how a system operates have been shown to be an important factor in reducing age differences in the speed and accuracy of decision making (Simon, 1968). The contemporary research of Rogers, Mayhorn, and Fisk (this volume) is based in part on the idea that the memory requirements of user interfaces for older users should utilize their long-term (semantic) memory because it is less affected by age-related cognitive decline than working memory.

The principle of optimal assignment of function to human and machine was provided in an informal analysis by Dr. John Senders. During the long debate about the wisdom of the Federal Aviation Administration age 60 limitation on pilots flying commercial passenger planes, several expert panels were convened to evaluate the ruling. Senders and I participated in one such group in 1985. After avowing that he knew nothing about aging, Dr. Senders discussed what he considered to be a poor assignment of function to pilot and computer. The result, he argued, was probably a greater risk to safety than health and functional risks associated with aging. His point was that advances in automatic aircraft control systems were continually reducing the human contribution of operating the aircraft to monitoring the system for low frequency malfunctions. Even experienced people can react inappropriately to rare, unexpected events. Senders argued that more active control of the aircraft should be given to the pilot and more of the performance monitoring for system malfunction to the computer system component.

APPLICATIONS TO AGING HELP HUMAN FACTORS AND GERONTOLOGY GROW UP RIGHT

HUMAN FACTORS ENGINEERING CONCEPTS BROADEN ECOLOGICAL CONCEPTS IN GERONTOLOGY

The thinking behind the applications of human factors to aging has also improved the articulation of the transactional or ecological model of person-environment relationships as represented in gerontology (Baltes & Baltes, 1990; Czaja, 1990a; Fozard & Popkin, 1978; Lawton, 1998; Lawton & Nahemow, 1973). For me, at least, the transactional view of person-environment relationships as articulated in human factors has provided a "world view" of aging that has guided much of my scientific work in gerontology (Fozard, 2000; Fozard, in press).

APPLICATIONS TO AGING BROADEN HUMAN FACTORS AND ERGONOMICS

The applications to aging have, in my opinion, significantly broadened the conceptual bases of human factors and ergonomics—an opinion reflected in the title of this epilogue. An important by-product of applying human factors to aging is an increased appreciation of individual differences among persons representing specific age cohorts at any one time, as well as the changes in the abilities, interests, and needs of individual persons in any age cohort as they age. Some specific impacts include the following:

- It reinforces a fundamental lesson of ergonomics that continuous secular changes over time, in the man-made environment, constantly reshape the dynamics of person-environment relationships. The ongoing developments of the new interdisciplinary field of gerontechnology (described by Bouma, 1992, 2001; Fozard, Graafmans, Rietsema, Bouma, & van Berlo, 1996; Fozard, Graafmans, Rietsema, van Berlo & Bouma, 1997; Fozard, Rietsema, Bouma, & Graafmans, 2000; and Graafmans, Fozard, Rietsema, van Berlo, & Bouma, 1994) over the past 15 years reflect the importance of this fundamental observation. The importance of changes within and between successive cohorts of aging persons for human factors engineering is also emphasized in the title (Gerotechnology) and contents of the present volume.
- The applications of human factors leading to an improved quality of life for older persons provide a useful guide to the field in general. In the National Research Council Report, research needs on functional abilities of elderly persons were identified in tasks related to transportation, home, workplace, leisure and safety and security (Czaja, 1990a). A similar contemporary scheme that relates areas of application to various tools or resources in research and engineering is described by van Bronswijk, Bouma, and Fozard (2003).
- Human factors research on aging has strengthened the interdisciplinary nature of the field by including a wider range of social science input, exemplified by chapters (this volume) by Mollenkopf on the social contexts of technology and Lesnoff-Caravaglia on ethical issues.
- The scope of human factors research has been broadened by the responses to the need for specific research related to aging. The National Research Council report on the human factors research

needs of an aging population cited three areas of need—distributional data on activities of older persons, task analyses of these activities, and ". . . direct contributions to the basic science of aging and behavior . . ." (Czaja, 1990b, pp. 59–67).

The remainder of this epilogue will discuss some of the developments highlighted above in relation to the present volume as well as some related published and anecdotal material.

PUTTING AGING AND SECULAR CHANGE
INTO THE PERSON/ENVIRONMENT MODEL

The analysis of age-related changes in a person's abilities and skills, as well as the secular changes in the environment in which aging occurs, increases the specificity of human factors. These additions suggest a modification of the traditional person/environment diagram as illustrated in Figure 17.1.

The traditional diagram has been modified in three ways. First, the components of the person part of the system have been divided into three components—receptors, internal states, and effectors—to permit better analysis of age-related changes in the human part of the system that affect system performance. Second, the environmental side has been divided into social, built, and natural or physical to permit better analyses of the importance of these components on system performance. Third, a time dimension has been added. It shows human aging and secular changes in the environment on the same scale. This dimension illustrates how different generations can have radically different experiences with particular man-machine systems that could affect their performance in system usage, e.g., different population stereotypes, etc.

The social science analyses relating successive age generations to secular changes in user interfaces (Sackmann & Weymaan, 1994; Mollenkopf, Meyer, Schultz, Wurm, & Friesdorf, 2000) have made a significant contribution to the understanding of the difficulties in, and motivation for, using technological products experienced by many older persons. The recent research on technology generations by Docampo Rama, deRidder, and Bouma (2001) specifically addressed this issue by comparing how well younger and older persons performed with menu-driven vs. electro-mechanical user interfaces. The main finding was that

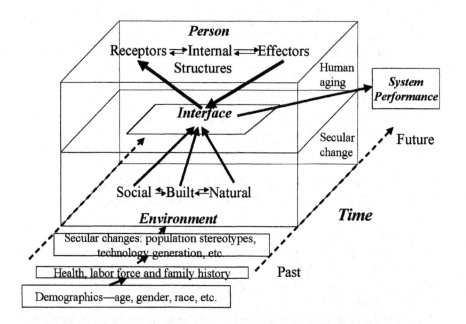

FIGURE 17.1 Diagram of dynamics of person/environment interface over time. The interaction of a person and the environment shows the three components of human response to environment that change with age (top half of figure), and the three components of the environment (built, social, physical or natural) that undergo secular change over time (lower half of figure). System performance is indicated by the box to the right of the diagram. Some antecedents contributing to the changing dynamics of the person/environment interface over time are shown in the boxes in the lower part of the figure. (Adapted from Fozard, 2002, in press).

individuals performed best on the interfaces that were most compatible with their own early experiences with technological products. As noted by Mollenkopf and Fozard (in press), we can expect the differences in secular changes in technology to create challenges to successive generations of older users. The implications of this person/environment dynamic on the motivation of older persons to utilize "new" technology are thoughtfully analyzed by Bouwhuis (2003). Ujimoto (this volume) examines the relationship between culture and locus of control in relation to the use of technical devices, including devices that serve as a substitute for humans in business transactions and information providing devices.

GREATER USER INVOLVEMENT IN PLANNING AND DESIGN PROCESSES

Two developments in gerontechnology cut across the work of human factors as related to aging (Bouma, 1992). The first is the idea of increasing user involvement in all phases of the development and distribution of technological products and environments. It is believed that this will reduce the trial and error aspects often observed in the development of new products and increase the market for new products. Also, it may reduce the stigma of products designed for "old people" (Bouma, 1992). The use of focus groups to elicit user input is described by Rogers, Meyers, Walker, and Fisk (1998) and Coleman (1998). Examples in the present volume include the chapters by Benbow and by Morrell, Mayhorn, and Echt, describing analyses of motivations and interests of older persons in relation to computer use.

The second development is the classification of application areas and the variety of approaches used to develop technology-based products, environments and services. This matrix of goals and means has evolved over a decade (Fozard, Rietsema, Graafmans, van Berlo, & Bouma, 1997) with the latest version described by van Bronswijk, Bouma, and Fozard (2003). One dimension of this matrix names the five domains of core ambitions of people ". . . most related to quality of life . . . health and self-esteem, mobility and transport, housing and living, communication and governance, and work and leisure" (p. 169). These domains of application are similar to those often used in health promotion models and to those listed in the National Research Council report mentioned earlier (Czaja, 1990b). The second dimension of the matrix lists four general ways in which technology can address the domains of applications:

- Enhancement and satisfaction, prevention and engagement, compensation and assistance, and care support and organization (p. 169).
- Enhancement and satisfaction refers to technology that increases the potential for self-expression and education, e.g., machines for creating or altering visual and auditory images, internet learning, etc. In the present volume, chapters by Benbow and by Smyth and Kwon exemplify this approach.
- Prevention and engagement refer primarily to the use of technology in early detection and prevention of illnesses and the support

of healthy lifestyles. Tran's chapter in the present volume exemplifies this concept.

- Compensation and assistance, and care support and organization, refer to applications that compensate for age-related functional decline and aid to caregivers of disabled elderly persons. Chapters related to this use of technology include those by Dienel, Cameron, and Peine, and by Watzke.

SOME MILESTONES IN THE DEVELOPMENT OF HUMAN FACTORS AND AGING

Dr. Chapanis' lecture on human factors engineering did not consider aging or human development. The major emphasis was on military applications, and most representatives of the systems' human component were in military uniform. One of the major contributors in the evolution of human factors and ergonomics was the spread into nonmilitary applications, a growth that continues vigorously today. The proliferation of technical interests groups (TIGs) in the Human Factors and Ergonomics Society reflected this evolution. Most of the initial TIGs were concerned with specialized areas of application, e.g., computer operations or special human functions, e.g., vision. The Technical Interest Group on Aging (TGA), initiated and nurtured by Dr. Arnold Small, was one of the first to focus on a class of people. Others were the Technical Interest Group on Personality and Individual Differences (TGPID) and the Technical Interest Group on Rehabilitation (TGR). With respect to the last named, it was originally proposed to have a single group focused on the elderly and disabled, a proposal that was properly rejected by both groups.

Promoting an interest in aging in the Society was a relatively slow process that took place in the 1970s and 1980s. I recall being the junior member of a small but enthusiastic group of scientists—Alan Welford, Ross McFarland, and MacElvaine Parsons, who, in various venues mostly organized by Dr. Small, made presentations on the importance of human factors in aging at meetings of the Society, the International Ergonomics Association, and Division 21 of the American Psychological Association (APA). Alphonse Chapanis wrote what I believe is the earliest article describing the relevance of human factors to gerontology in a publication of the Gerontological Society of America (Chapanis, 1974). My invited address to the APA's Division 21 culminated in a paper with Sam

Popkin (Fozard & Popkin, 1978), and Ross McFarland and I put together the first special edition on Human Factors (Fozard, 1981), a project repeated a decade later under the editorship of Sara Czaja (1990b).

It took several years for the TGA to become a stable group. During the four years I served as TGA chair, most of our sessions were attended by Dr. Small, the speakers, and a very small group of interested members, sometimes including James Baker, who also served as TGA chair for a year. It was not until 1989 that there were enough members that a legitimate election of officers could take place, resulting in the election of Sara Czaja as chair of the TGA.

Since the 1980s the pace of activity and interest in human factors related to aging has accelerated dramatically. The development of gerontechnology as a discipline during the 1990s established a broader context for human factors, ergonomics, and aging than was common at the time (Bouma, 2001; Fozard, 2002). Specifically, it dealt with the issues of decision-making and advocacy in the development and distribution of technology for older people, the role of the consumer in designing technology, and the specifics of the integration of engineering sciences with gerontology and its components—biology, psychology, and sociology. The creation of the International Society for Gerontechnology, the journal *Gerontechnology*, the four international conferences on gerontechnology and the publication of their proceedings (Bouma & Graafmans, 1992; Graafmans, Taipele, & Charness, 1998; Pieper, Vaarma, & Fozard, 2003; Charness, Czaja, Fisk, & Rogers, 2002), and the textbook on gerontechnology edited by Harrington and Harrington (2000) have provided a solid basis and a broad context for human factors and ergonomics as applied to aging.

In the U.S., the establishment of a Special Interest Group on Technology and Aging (TAG) in the Gerontological Society of America increased awareness of the significance of technology and aging and the importance of human factors and ergonomics. This has been most obvious since S. Kwon became the convener of the Group. Using the Internet, Kwon has also spearheaded a very broad-based international interest group called Gerotechnology.

Many of the persons who have contributed to *Gerontechnology* are also involved in current efforts in gerotechnology, e.g., Charness & Schaie (2003). The contents of the present volume reflect this broad base. The publication of the *Handbook of Human Factors and Aging* (Fisk & Rogers, 1997), and the advances in and ever-sharper distinctions between universal design and design for specific disabilities (Coleman & Myerson,

2001) have made important contributions to the current developments of human factors and ergonomics related to aging.

In conclusion, the present volume provides an excellent overview of the international scope of current applications of human factors and aging, provided by what I estimate to be the third to fifth generation of an international group of scientists and practitioners. Writing this epilogue resulted in my developing a list of earlier major publications related to the development of ergonomics and human factors as discussed here. I have mentioned some of the publications, but offer the following list in Table 17.1 as the ones that represent important developmental markers. It is by no means complete, and I apologize in advance to colleagues for any significant errors. The titles and references are given in the references. The table headings indicate the *author and year of publication*, and the major role(s) their work played in developing the field—*define issues, broaden scope of field, tell others in gerontology about human factors and ergonomics as related to aging.*

TABLE 17.1 Important Publications in the Development of Human Factors and Aging Related to Aging

Author, Year of publication	Define Issues	Broaden Scope	Tell Other Players
Welford, 1956	X		X
Chapanis, 1974	X		X
Fozard & Popkin, 1978	X	X	X
Fozard, 1981, Czaja, 1990	X	X	
Czaja, 1990 (NRC Rep.)	X	X	X
Charness & Bosman, 1990	X		X
Fozard, Graafmans, Rietsema, Bouma,& van Berlo (1996) Bouma, 2001*	X	X	X
Fisk & Rogers, 1997	X	X	
Harrington & Harrington, 2000	X	X	X
Coulson, 2000		X	X
Sagawa & Bouma, 2001	X	X	
Burdick & Kwon, 2005	X	X	X

* Summarizes numerous publications.

ACKNOWLEDGMENTS

James L. Fozard is affiliated with Florida Gerontological Research and Training Services, 2980 Tangerine Terrace, Palm Harbor, FL 34684-4039. E-mail: fozard@knology.net

REFERENCES

Baltes, P. B., & Baltes, M. M. (1990). Psychological perspectives on successful aging: The model of selective optimization with compensation. In P. B. Baltes & M. M. Baltes (Eds.), *Successful aging: Perspectives from the behavioral sciences* (pp. 1–34). Cambridge: Cambridge University Press.

Bouma, H. (1992). Gerontechnology: A framework on technology and aging. In H. Bouma & J. A. M. Graafmans (Eds.), *Gerontechnology* (pp. 1–7). Amsterdam: IOS Press.

Bouma, H. & Graafmans, A. M. (Eds.) (1992). *Gerontechnology.* Amsterdam: IOS Press.

Bouma, H. (2001). Editorial. *Gerontechnology, 1*(1), 1–3.

Bouwhuis, D. G. (2003). Design for person-environment interaction in older age: A gerontechnological perspective. *Gerontechnology, 2,* 231–246.

Burdick, D. C. & Kwon, S. (Eds.) (2005). *Gerotechnology: Research and practice in technology and aging.* New York: Springer Publishing.

Chapanis, A. (1974). Human engineering environments for the aged. *Gerontologist, 6,* 228–235.

Chapanis, A., & McCollum, I. A. (1956). *Joint services annotated bibliography of human factors in design.* San Diego State College Foundation, Contract Nonr-1968.

Charness, N., & Bosman, E. A. (1990). Human factors and design for older adults. In J. E. Birren & K. W. Schaie (Eds.), *Handbook of the psychology of aging* (3rd ed.). New York: Academic Press.

Charness, N., & Schaie, K. W. (Eds.) (2003). *Impact of technology on successful aging.* New York: Springer Publishing.

Charness, N., Czaja, S., Fisk, A. D., & Rogers, W. A. (Eds.) (2002). Congress issue: Gerontechnology 2002. *Gerontechnology, 2*(1), 1–155.

Coleman, R. (1998). Improving the quality of life for older people by design. In J. A. M. Graafmans, V. Taipele, & N. Charness (Eds.), *Gerontechnology: A sustainable investment in the future* (pp. 74—83). Amsterdam: IOS Press.

Coleman, R., & Myerson, J. (2001). Improving life quality by countering design exclusion. *Gerontechnology, 2*(1), 88–102.

Coulson, I. (Ed.) (2000). Special issue: Technological challenges for gerontologists in the 21st century. *Educational Gerontology, 26*(4), 307–316.

Czaja, S. J. (Ed.) (1990a). *Human factors needs for an aging population*. Washington, DC: National Academy Press.

Czaja, S. J. (Ed.) (1990b). Special issue on aging. *Human Factors, 32*.

Docampo Rama, M., de Ridder, H., & Bouma, H. (2001). Technology generation and age in using layered interfaces. *Gerontechnology, 1*(1), 25–40.

Fisk, A. D., & Rogers, W. A. (Eds.) (1997). *Handbook of human factors and the older adult*. San Diego, CA: Academic Press.

Fozard, J. L (Ed.) 1981. *Special Issue: Aging. Human Factors*, 23(1), 1–124.

Fozard, J. L. (2000). How ten years with ageless rats and college sophomores led to a thirty-something year career in geropsychology. In. J. E. Birren & J. H. H. Schroots (Eds.), *History of geropsychology through autobiography* (pp. 91–108). Washington, DC: American Psychological Association.

Fozard, J. L. (2002). Gerontechnology: Beyond ergonomics and universal design. *Gerontechnology, 1*(3), 137–139.

Fozard, J. L. (in press) Gerontechnology: Optimizing relationships between aging people and changing technology. In I. C. Coulson & V. Minichiello (Eds.), *Contemporary issues in gerontology: Promoting positive ageing*. Sydney: Allen & Unwin.

Fozard, J. L., & Popkin, S. J. (1978). Optimizing adult development: Ends and means of an applied psychology of aging. *American Psychologist, 33,* 975–989.

Fozard, J. L., Graafmans, J. A. M., Rietsema, J., Bouma, H., & van Berlo, A. (1996). Aging and ergonomics: The challenges of individual differences and environmental change. In K. Brookhuis, C. Weikert, J. Moraal, & D. de Waard, (Eds.), *Aging and human factors* (pp. 51–66). Groningen, The Netherlands: TRC, University of Groningen.

Fozard, J. L., Graafmans, J. A. M., Rietsema, J., van Berlo, G. M. W., & Bouma, H. (1997). Gerontechnology: Technology to improve health, functioning and quality of life of aging and aged adults. *Korean Journal of Gerontology, 7*(1), 110–122.

Fozard, J. L., Rietsema, J., Bouma, H., & Graafmans, J. A. M. (2000). Gerontechnology: Creating enabling environments for the challenges and opportunities of aging. *Educational Gerontology, 26,* 331–334.

Graafmans, J. A. M., Fozard, J. L., Rietsema, J., van Berlo, A., & Bouma, H. (1994). Gerontechnology: A sustainable development in society. In G. Wild & A. Kirschner (Eds.), *Safety-alarm systems, technical aids and smart homes* (pp. 9–24). Knegsel, The Netherlands: Akontes.

Graafmans, J. A. M., Taipele, V., & Charness, N. (Eds.) (1998). *Gerontechnology: A sustainable investment in the future*. Amsterdam: IOS Press.

Harrington, T. L., & Harrington, M. K. (2000). *Gerontechnology: Why and how*. Maastricht, The Netherlands: Shaker Press.

Lawton, M. P. (1998). Future society and technology. In J. A. M. Graafmans, V. Taipele, & N. Charness (Eds.), *Gerontechnology: A sustainable investment in the future* (pp. 12–22). Amsterdam: IOS Press.

Lawton, M. P., & Nahemow, L. (1973). Ecology and the aging process. In C. Eisdorfer & M. P. Lawton (Eds.), *The psychology of adult development and aging.* Washington, DC: American Psychological Association.

Lockard, R. B., & Fozard, J. L. (1956). The eye as a control mechanism. Navy Ordnance Testing Station, NOTS Rep. 1046, August, 1956.

Mollenkopf, H., Meyer, S., Schulz, E., Wurm, S., & Friesdorf, W. (2000). Technik im Haushalt zur Unterstützung einer selbstbestimmten Lebensfuhrung im Alter: Das Forschungsproject "sentha" und erste Ergebnisse des sozialwissenschaftlichen Teilprojekts. *Zeitschrift für Gerontologie und Geriatrie, 33(3),* 155–168.

Mollenkopf, H., & Fozard, J. L. (2004). Technology and the good life: Challenges for current and future generations of aging people. In H-W. Wahl, R. Scheidt, & P. Windley (Eds.), *Environments, gerontology and old age: Annual review of gerontology and geriatrics* (pp. 250–279). New York: Springer Publishing.

Pieper, R., Vaarama, M., & Fozard, J. L. (Eds.) (2003). *Gerontechnology: Technology and aging: Starting into the third millennium.* Aachen, Germany: Shaker Verlag.

Rogers, W. A., Meyers, B., Walker, N., & Fisk, A. D. (1998). Functional limitations to daily living tasks in the aged: A focus group analysis. *Human Factors, 40,* 111–125.

Sackmann, A., & Weymann, A. (1994). *Die Technisierung des Altags: Generationen und technische Innovationen* [The technization of everyday life. Generations and technical innovations] Frankfurt: Campus.

Sagawa, K., & Bouma, H. (Eds.) (2001). *Proceedings of the International Workshop on Gerontechnology.* National Institute of Bioscience and Human-Technology, Tsukuba, Japan, March 2001.

Simon, J. R. (1968). Signal processing time as a function of aging. *Journal of Experimental Psychology, 78,* 76–80.

Steenbekkers, L. P. A., & van Beijsterveldt, C. E. M. (Eds.) (1998). *Design-relevant characteristics of ageing users.* Delft, The Netherlands: Delft University Press.

van Bronswijk, J. E. M. H., Bouma, H., & Fozard, J. L. (2003). Technology for quality of life: An enriched taxonomy. *Gerontechnology, 2(2),* 169–172.

Subject Index

Page numbers followed by *f* indicate figures. Those followed by *t* indicate tables.

Springer Publishing Company

Annual Review of Gerontology and Geriatrics, *Volume 23*

Aging in Context: Socio-Physical Environments

Hans-Werner Wahl, PhD, Rick J. Scheidt, PhD, and Paul G. Windley, PhD, Volume Editors

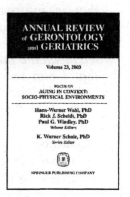

In this volume dedicated to M. Powell Lawton, the editors emphasize the need to create new bridges to connect research studies focusing on objective physical environments and other studies mainly addressing subjective person-environment components.

Partial Contents:

- The General Ecological Model Revisited: Evolution, Current Status, and Continuing Challenges, *R.J. Scheidt and L. Norris-Baker*
- Ecology and the Aging Self, *R.L. Rubinstein and K. de Medeiros*
- Assessing the Fit Between Older People and Their Home Environments— An Occupational Therapy Research Perspective, *S. Iwarsson*
- Socio-Physical Environments at the Macro Level: The Impact of Population Migration, *C.F. Longino*
- Everyday Competence and Everyday Problem Solving in Aging Adults: Role of the Physical and Social Context, *M. Diehl and S.L. Willis*
- Interior Living Environments in the Adult Life Course, *G.D. Rowles, F. Oswald, and E. Hunter*
- Correlates of Residential Satisfaction in Adulthood and Old Age: A Meta-Analysis, *M. Pinquart and D. Burmedi*
- Neighborhood, Health, and Well-Being in Late Life, *N. Krause*
- Technology and the Good Life: Challenges for Current and Future Generations of Aging People, *H. Mollenkopf and J.L. Fozard*
- The Urban-Rural Distinction in Gerontology, *S.M. Golant*

2004 400pp 0-8261-1734-1 hardcover

11 West 42nd Street, New York, NY 10036-8002 • Fax: 212-941-7842
Order Toll-Free: 877-687-7476 • Order On-line: www.springerpub.com

CPSIA information can be obtained
at www.ICGtesting.com
Printed in the USA
BVOW11*2252110416

443809BV00005B/15/P